AF326653

Food's Tree of Paradise

Food's Tree of Paradise

R. Shelton, CLMT, BCTMB

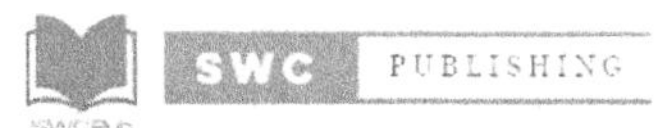

Arizona, Published 2024, First Edition

Copyright © 2024 R. Shelton, Clinically Licensed Massage Therapist, Board Certification in Therapeutic Massage and Bodywork

Cover: R. Shelton, CLMT, BCTMB
Photograph: Webvilla
All rights reserved. Some names and identifying details have been changed to protect the privacy of individuals.

NOTE: "*Food's Tree of Paradise*" reflects only the personal experience and views of the author. The information contained in this book is for educational purposes only. The author of this book does not dispense medical advice or prescribe the use of any technique as a form of treatment for physical or medical problems without the advice of a physician, either directly or indirectly. The intent of the author is only to offer information of a general nature to help you in your quest for physical, emotional, and spiritual well-being. In the event you use any of the information in this book for yourself, which is your constitutional right, the author and the publisher assume no responsibility for your actions. Proper care from a physician should not be avoided, delayed, or discarded when there is reason to consult a physician. Conditions requiring proper medical attention should be referred to a physician.   – R. Shelton

Hardcover ISBN: 978-0-9998586-7-7

First printing: 2024
Printed in the United States of America
SWC Publishing.
Available Anywhere Books Are Sold
Library of Congress Catalog Card Number:
Paperback ISBN: 978-0-9998586-8-4
In E-Book: ISBN: 978-0-9998586-9-1

"I rise in the morning, and I eat.

I rise from my labors, and I eat.

I rise all the day,

I rise all the night,

All my life I rise to eat,

And my food eats me."

- R. Shelton

Acknowledgements

I will always thank my Creator for showing me the way to free myself from the shackles of the slavery to food that I hadn't even realized were there not just in my life but in all our lives. Like in any discipline, what we eat is another area over which we can gain self-control and mastery. I am grateful for the liberty that my being can enjoy as I follow the basic principles of eating in a more healthy and balanced way of living life with food in it; it brings me more joy and strength.

Next, I thank my husband, who is supportive of my hopes, my dreams, and most of all my seemingly never-ending writing process with all these new books. He's a trooper!

Many thanks to my clients for all you have taught me, for your support, and inspiration. Each one of you has touched my life in one way or another.

Last but not least, I thank *you*. Thank you for reading and reviewing this book, for having the courage to try new things, and for hoping for a better tomorrow by improving the things you do today. You make a difference in the world, and I'm so glad that you are in it. May you find inspiration in these pages and new ways to take action on this resource.

Contents

Chapter 1
Food Wars

FOOD'S TREE OF PARADISE

HELPLESS AND HOPELESS, prisoners to food, many people are enslaved to addictive ingredients, food-combining patterns set in place by family and caregivers, social media, and friends and enemies alike - set in place for so long no one even remembers there *was* a Food Tree of Paradise. Today, many prefer to falsely believe that foods do not affect or change the body's overall chemistry or affect its health. But they do. Not only is my life living proof of this evidence, but science also clearly supports the fact that foods *do indeed* matter and create various chemical reactions within the body.

Food can slowly kill you or lead the body to a much more robust life. I want you to think about it this way, even if you currently do not believe this. Just humor me for a short bit while I explain how it works; assume I'm right. At least be curious enough to explore why I'm presenting this information in the way that I am. If by the end of the book you find you don't agree, just go back to your own ideas.

Each and every day, there is a war going on inside your body, and the struggle for power hangs in the balance. Who will win depends on *you* and what you choose to put inside it. Are you giving communication and supplies to the enemy? Who *is* this enemy? The enemy consists of bad bacteria, parasites, and things that destroy the telomeres [*] like stress, our thoughts, and emotions. Additionally, improper balance of foods creates so much acidity in the body that it can cause the red blood cells to explode and release internal acidity into the bloodstream. This, in turn, causes cravings for *more* acidic foods, which then affect even *more* blood cells, causing them to explode and die, releasing more and more acid.

There was a tent-maker by the name of Paul who lived in a very large, wealthy town that was bordered by two harbors. You can imagine the influx of merchants and trade going on daily as well as the hustle and bustle of life - and all with every ideology under the sun. In this city, there were many indulgences going on including the residents and some of the Corinthians engaging in the worship of idols. Paul, an apostle of Jesus Christ, condemned this. As he touched on the topic, he first prepared their minds with this concept [1] that relates, interestingly, to the topic of foods. The topic was that if any man loves God, that person is known by God.

Here, Paul references the massive engagement in idol worship and the sacrifices given to idols. He says that we know that we all have knowledge about these things.

Knowledge puffs people up, he says, but true, Christ-like love edifies. He continues by saying that anyone who thinks he knows anything really knows nothing yet, at least not the way he ought to know it.

Knowledge puffs people up.

It is too easy to read something, to learn a thing from whatever source, and to believe that we know all there is to know on the matter. It is a common phenomenon that involves the ego. Once we get something in our minds, it creates a pathway—a groove, and the concept swells each time we review it, as if it has swollen up so tightly that there is no room remaining for any new or additional information.

It's not that there's *not* any room, it's just that it takes too much work to change, add to, or completely overhaul it for more information that may actually be even better, more accurate, or even more helpful than what we've already got. At least, it feels... too hard.

According to *Psychology Today* [**], cognitive dissonance is that uncomfortable feeling you get when two modes of thought contradict each other. Clashing conditions may include ideas, beliefs, or the knowledge that one has behaved in a certain way.

The theory of cognitive dissonance suggests that people are against feeling inconsistencies within their own minds. It explains why people will go out of their way to shift their thinking when their own words, thoughts, or behaviors seem to clash with each other. This helps them *feel* better about *not* changing their minds to be more in alignment with actual truth.

Why do we do this? Fear of the unknown.

Even when the unknown, while scary *at first*, has potential to help us feel better than we ever have before, it's the fear that we might feel *worse* (than we ever have before) that stops us. The *fear* that we'll lose the rose-colored glasses we've dreamed up causes us to live in inside our own minds. Each person has their own perception of what life is like and how everyone else moves within it and around them. This fear can be so intense that we can that we may even convince ourselves we don't hear or see the opposing idea(s) at all.

If change and self-improvement is actually such a good thing and is truly desirable, there *has* to be a way to work around this. Good news: there is!

One way to avoid cognitive dissonance when things don't fit together may include denying or compartmentalizing unwelcomed thoughts, putting them in their own separate mental box for a bit while you get more comfortable with taking an honest look at them at a safer time.

Another way people tend to deal with conflicting ideas is to look for a way to explain away a thought that doesn't seem to fit with the others. For example, try asking yourself: what else could this mean?

A third option is to be willing and open to change your belief or behavior. This last option can certainly help to "de-puff" knowledge and allow space for true Christ-like love to enter. We can let go of false beliefs or ideas that don't truly serve us and make room for new, better behaviors and/or concepts to reside within us.

Living in the lie that is cognitive dissonance is akin to this never-ending downward spiral of acid breeding more acid, like with our telomeres. It's only going to increase the advantage that the bad bacteria and parasites have over the good bacteria inside our bodies. It's in the bad bacteria's best interest to keep you feeling warm, cozy, and familiar with the way *they* like things. Indeed, there is definitely some mind control at work as well.

The science community has proven parasite and bacteria's abilities to metaphorically blind you to just how much the body is falling apart internally. That's how they like it. Get that balanced with foods, and, wow! You'll be surprised how much more self-control you'll have and how much better you'll feel too! Every choice you make comes down to feeding your acid-state/bad bacteria or for providing nourishment and filling sources of supplies that will strengthen the body's defense system.

Overnourishing the body can be just as much of a problem and can likewise become destructive if it gets too much power as well. A recurring theme in my first two books, *"Member Heal Thyself"* and *"Fountain of Living Water"* is that balance in *all* things is vital to a long lasting life.

In his first letter to the church in Thessalonica, the capital city of Macedonia at the time and named in honor of Thessalonica, sister of Alexander the Great and wife of the Greek military leader Cassander, Paul writes and urges the people to be full of light.

There is an actual, literal difference that can be physically seen in a person's countenance, in their face, between a person who is eating "clean" and one who is not.

The one eating "clean" is filled with light. Those who do not, have a dark cast to their skin, a dullness, greyish-ness, or even a green-sickly color.

To drive the point home about how important taking care of what we put in and on our bodies, let's interject some history from the Native American tribes.

For simplicity's sake, we'll divide the Native Americans into two groups, though there were many tribes involved and intermingled. The first group loved to destroy, enslave, and take advantage, and the second group loved life, liberty, and family. This is very similar to the bacteria in our bodies. There are bacteria that build our health and bacteria that destroy it and damage tissues and organs.

The leader of the people of light had a vision of the future. The vision would come to pass four hundred years from the time Christ had appeared to their people after his crucifixion and resurrection. In the vision, the leader saw that the people would dwindle in unbelief. He gave his son his position so he could go and teach the people and strengthen their hearts in hopes of preventing this from happening. He told his son about the vision but charged him not to tell anyone about his dream.

What the leader saw coming were wars, pestilence, famine, and bloodshed—even to the point that their group of good tribes would become extinct. He told his son in the vision he saw that the reason this could happen was because the people were going to fall into works of darkness, all manner of lusts, and evil doings.

His son also took up the cause to teach the people after his father passed away. But there were many who would not listen to him and instead loved the work of destruction. These people wanted someone else to be in charge; and they wanted a king instead.

The man they had in mind was a large, strong man by the name of Amalickiah, and Amalickiah's *desire* was to be king. He was part of the greater number of the people and had gotten a position as one of the lower judges of the land (kind of similar to America's district court), and these lower judges wanted *power*.

Amalickiah flattered the other lower judges, telling them that if they supported him in becoming king, then he would make them rulers over the people, even though these judges were also being reinforced with good teachings by their *true* leader and *even* though they were the *high priests* of the church!

Fast forwarding a bit, Amalickiah wrought great destruction among his own people—the people of light—and then planned to go over to the tribes who loved bloodshed and darkness and become their leader so he could strengthen his numbers. But a very good, righteous man, a powerful military leader, saw what was going on began to gather together and stir up the hearts of the people of light who believed in maintaining balance and order and goodness in the land to defend and protect their liberty.

Amalickiah knew that if he was caught and taken to court that he and the group following him would be charged and found guilty of tyranny. He knew that what he was up to was not just or right. So, he fled to the dark tribes and used treachery, murder, and intrigue against them to become *their* king. Thus, he gained his design to have power over them, and those men and judges were even more ferocious and evil than the dark-hearted tribes.

It was part of Amalickiah's plan to gain control over the part of this dark kingdom, that favored their own king. And so, he tricked the king into putting Amalickiah in charge of his dark army. The next part of the plan was to make the dark tribes angry so they would want to go destroy the good tribes who believed in goodness and light, (from where he had just come).

There was just one little problem with this plan: some members of the king's army were *afraid* of displeasing the king, but they were *also* afraid to go up to battle against the good tribes, especially since they had only recently lost a war to the people of light. They feared they would lose their lives if they went to battle again. Most of the army refused to go into battle again.

The king of the dark tribes became very angry at this and that was when he put Amalickiah in charge. Amalickiah took the obedient members of the army and tried to force the rest of the army to take up arms. Remember, his *true* desire was to dethrone the king and become king himself.

The members of the army who refused to fight all ran away and hid themselves in a place called Onidah, known as the place of arms. There they appointed a third man to be their king and a leader over them, determined they would not be forced to go to battle against the good tribes.

The part of the army hidden away at Onidah went to the mountain to prepare to defend themselves against their brothers. What they didn't realize was that Amalickiah never intended to fight them. He just wanted the original king and the obedient part of the army to think so.

See, if Amalickiah got control of the entire army he would be able to dethrone the king and take possession of the entire kingdom. He brought his little army to the base of the mountain in a nearby valley and set up camp there. When night fell, he sent a secret embassy up into the mountain asking the leader there to come down to the foot of the mountain to talk with him.

(Let us just pause here for a moment from our vantage point of knowing what's in the hearts of all the parties involved here and shout out together to the leader at Onidah, *"DON'T GO!!!"*)

Good news: the Onidah leader did *not* go down to the foot of the mountain! He knew if he did, he would lose his safe position and advantage and his army would not be able to help if and when things got hinky. Plus, he knew that Amalickiah was up to no-good.

Amalickiah asked a second time for the Onidah leader to come down to the foot of the mountain, and the leader would not come. Amalickiah invited him again a third time to come down. But he still would not come.

Finally, Amalickiah got the message: this guy is not going to come down to the foot of the mountain. Instead, Amalickiah himself went up the mountain, nearly to the leader's camp and asked him to meet Amalickiah—he could even bring his guards with him!

(Can I just say: never agree to a deal, even just a conversation, with anyone who is not in agreement with your wellness goals. It will never end well, especially not for you.)

Amalickiah convinced the leader that he wanted the leader and his men to come down during the night and surround Amalickiah's men in their camps, and Amalickiah would deliver the king's army into the leader's hands on the condition that as long as he would make Amalakiah the leader's second in command over the whole army.

The Onidah leader believed this, even though it was a trick, and he put Amalakiah in charge under himself. Then, Amalakiah slowly poisoned the leader to death and gained control of the entire army himself. Then he could dethrone the original king, gain possession over the entire kingdom, and go to battle against his own people—the people of light—and take possession of *their* lands too.

From this example we can see how quickly darkness and sickness can spread.

When the people (or the good bacteria) are not strong and filled with light and wisdom, they are quickly and easily overtaken. In the story, the people of light became dark and were utterly destroyed from off the face of the land, eventually overrun and murdered by the dark tribes under Amalickiah's hand. Archeologists are now uncovering the remains of these civilizations and evidence of these wars. It's not just a story of the war of an ancient people but also a warning of the delicate battle going on within our bodies.

If you are not aware of food choices you make and decide to eat however you feel is fine, or right to eat, you could *already* be falling into the dark, as Paul calls it. Though knowledge puffs us up, and we are asleep to *real* information, Paul urges us in his letter that real information could awaken us and fill our countenances with light. We should not sleep as others do.

Paul tells the people of Thessalonica—and us—to watch together and to be sober and abstain from partaking of things that hurt or destroy. [2] He creates a visual representation of wearing protective armor, which proper nutrition can bring internally and externally. We can take action in love with hope in our hearts for good nutrition's ability to help save us and, in this case, prevent many health problems.

Creating balance in the body is not a firm line in the sand, which can make it trickier to figure out the right foods to eat. Why is this? Each person has a unique make up; we each have different susceptibilities and weaknesses in our own bodies, different triggers, life-length time tables. No one is the same as any other person; not even twins.

Take Hezekiah, for example. He was king of Judah and was a great religious and political reformer, as it is told. He had the help of the prophet Isaiah, and the early part of his reign was prosperous. Some of the things he did and the types of interactions and conflicts he must have been dealing with were surely intense.

At this point of his story, we find him sick almost to the point of death. [3] (If you're familiar with my story, which I shared a bit of in "*Member Heal Thyself*" this part really hits home for me, having almost died due to illness myself.) The prophet Isaiah even went to Hezekiah and told him that he needed to get his house in order because he was going to die for sure.

The king was devastated. It's one thing to *feel* like you're dying but quite another to have someone called to come tell you it's a done deal, that you're *going* to die. It's not just in your head. He was such a good person, and he was going to die. There were a lot of other factors to Hezekiah's story, but I'm not going to dive into that here.

We all have different weaknesses in our bodies. A person's body is usually the first place that we notice that disaster strikes. There are as many illnesses as there are people in the world, with many root causes, and as many solutions. Even back when Jesus was living on the earth, he went all over Galilee [4] teaching the simplified pure gospel in the synagogues and churches, healing all manner of sickness, and performing miracles. He went about curing all manner of diseases among the people who believed in him. A world full of illness is not a new thing, nor is healing. Part of healing can be done through the foods we eat. Most dis-ease cannot thrive in a balanced and wholesome body.

Signs of physical imbalance show up first in the smallest muscles of the body, even in our cells, and in already damaged areas like where we've previously inured ourselves. Even if the wounds have mostly healed and we don't notice them as much, negative emotions may still be trapped in the tissue—even spiritual trauma of which we may be completely unaware.

Until we take care of all three aspects of the wellness triangle (see Figure 1.),—the physical, mental/emotional, and the spiritual—for that injury, it will never fully heal. And very much like an infected sliver that we mostly cleaned out (leaving the rest to take care of itself), that infection is going to return and probably end up worse than it was initially. It may cause further and sometimes worse, possibly more dangerous, complications.

Overcoming trials and adversity in life cannot happen without proper nutrients in the body to strengthen it. If a soldier going to war is starving or has been malnourished for a while, he will not be able to cope with the physical and emotional stressors he will face. In fact, this may be so much—too much—that he may not survive mentally or emotionally intact. This does not mean only physical food but also spiritual food, mental/emotional food: food for the body, heart, and mind.

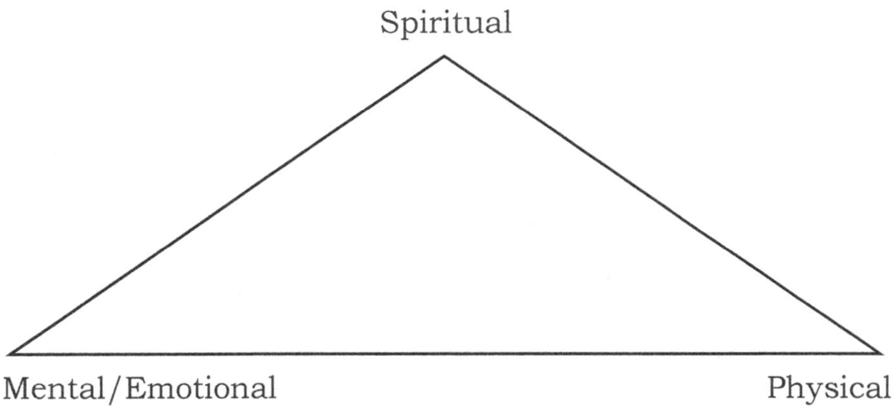

Figure 1. The Wellness Triangle

FOOD'S TREE OF PARADISE

Chapter 2
Fran: Cancer

IN MY LIFE AND MUCH of my working career, I have seen people of all ages who have walked through experiencing cancer in their lives. My own family has had more than its fair share. In my immediate family, my grandmother, mother, and two of my sisters all had cancer. Two survived; two did not.

I have seen the life-long devastation cancer can cause—the cruel side-effects of the treatments, and not just on the person with cancer but also each individual in the family. I've watched those on the outskirts, wishing they could help, not knowing how, and wind up choosing to do nothing because they didn't know where to begin looking for where to start.

In the last two decades, the world has seen a rise in support groups and fundraisers to try and boost morale of caregivers and help pay the overwhelming bills in the face of decreased income and rise in the cost of patient care more so than any other illness, it seems.

The damage that something as tremendous and destructive as cancer can cause—when the body can no longer control its own cell growth through natural means—can be life-altering. For one woman I met—I'll call her Fran—it was epiphanic.

Fran told me she had never really wanted to have children. No, let me restate: she *never* wanted to have kids. *Ever.* Her life-style reflected this in every aspect; there were no inconsistencies in her life in regard to this matter. She enjoyed occasionally stepping into the role of aunt but that was the hard line stop of it. Maybe using the word *enjoyed* in the full sense of the word was taking things too far. She enjoyed the carefree life of eating out several times a week at restaurants, staying up late, drinking, etc., and she never wanted to change her lifestyle, seeing no harm in it.

One day, Fran said, she wasn't feeling very well. This had been going on for a *little* bit of time, so, like any responsible woman somewhat in tune with her body, she decided to make an appointment with her primary care physician. Like so many others, Fran was not prepared for the diagnosis she received, probably expecting that she had caught some bacterial infection or a bad case of the flu.

I'd like to pause a moment at this point in the story to point out the importance and meaning of the term "disease" (origin: *disease* means "lack of *ease*"), and it's three-point cocktail. That would be the matter of timing of an insult, our thoughts and their contribution to helping brew a perfect storm, and toxicity. The combination of these three principles all at the same time can lead to incredible destruction within the body. See if you can spot all three in Fran's story.

You see, when the doctor came back and told Fran that she had cancer—and not only cancer, but a very aggressive and fast-growing form of it—in her mind she thought it was an acute condition. *Acute* means that it is just newly happening. Like falling and breaking your arm or getting hit by a car or something kind of new. But this was not the case at all.

Nutritionally, there is usually long-term malnutrition occurring that results in the bones not being as strong and hard as they normally could and should be. Bones are not completely solid as most of us have been led to believe. They're more sponge-like and more of a thick, very slow liquid that can slowly bend and curve over time. Preferably they stay straight, but I have seen it for myself. Also when the bones are weak and brittle, they break much more easily than when they are strong and healthy.

From a nutritional standpoint, Fran was not standing on solid ground. Her lascivious lifestyle had her consuming large quantities of acid-forming foods. Being in her life's early stage, she had enough life force in her body's wellness warehouse to borrow against so as not to consciously notice the affects until that point. How she had chosen to live her life—with each bit of food she put in her mouth, each sip of wine, and coffee she enjoyed in excess of what her body could actually handle—had finally caught up to her.

Too much meat, too many bad carbs and processed foods, and not enough other things to help her body rest, cleanse, and nourish her cells and organs. There were so many assaults on her body nutritionally that it didn't stand a chance to create balance. Her body got further and further behind "being healthy" that eventually it couldn't catch up.

Toxicity years in the making. The garbage in Fran's body kept piling up and piling up. And we all know what happens when you leave garbage sitting around. It starts to smell worse and worse and releases harmful gasses. Imagine if you could never air that out, ever, and you're living inside it. Eventually you go nose blind to it and stop noticing it. You may even falsely believe there's no problem and keep doing what you've been doing. And perhaps you won't even believe it if other people tell you they see (*or smell*) a problem!

Here comes good old cognitive dissonance puffing up our own knowledge and blocking our ears from hearing or taking in any new information that is contrary or the opposite of what we want to believe.

I'm always a bit curious about illness and its origins. Sometimes things are truly just genetic. No way around that. Many times, things can be tied back to a bad experience, an imbalance of some sort. These things are much easier to work with much of the time, if a person is willing to resolve and reverse the situation.

I had a conversation with Fran about her situation with cancer, and this led us to a deeper dive into her life before the dis-ease showed up. Initially, she insisted that there had been no emotionally triggering events for her. However, I had a hunch that there had been *something,* and I persisted in exploring the line of conversation further.

Still insisting there was absolutely nothing unresolved in her life, I left her with a suggestion: it was most likely some event that had held a very strong emotion for her, good or bad, that she had perhaps attempted to brush off as nothing or sweep under the rug. I asked her to allow herself to be open enough to at least consider the possibility.

I don't recall if a day or a week had passed, but Fran called me back with urgency in her voice. There *had* been an event! She had quite forgotten it, but during the event she had become extremely upset over the matter. It had to do with a relationship she had been in, but was no longer. She had moved on in her life and thought it was over. Subconsciously, though, her mind and heart had stewed on it because there had been no successful resolution reached, no apologies made, and no restitution.

The situation had been so emotionally devastating to her heart that she consciously could not bear it. She took the first step—as all other options had become unavailable to her in this situation she could see to take as all other options had become unavailable to her in this situation— she had to get herself somewhere safe. So, she left the emotionally toxic environment that was causing her so much unbearable pain. To her conscious mind, she had escaped; the threat was over! To protect her from how *extra* everything was, her mind had hidden away the rest of what she actually had not been able to handle. And it got stored away in her body to deal with and take care of later!

But she didn't take care of it.

Because Fran felt so much relief at the momentary escape of the emotionally toxic situation and her subconscious brain did such a great job hiding it from her awareness, she mistakenly thought, that everything was done, over, and gone. Completely!

Her body tried to get her attention in little ways to let her know there was still work that needed to be done. She needed to finish releasing the emotional trauma but her conscious mind stubbornly fought for control of this falsely created rose-colored world in which she now lived. In this safe world, things like what had happened to her did not exist.

She began to become more controlling of everyone around her. She did not realize it herself until quite a long time later in her healing process when it was safe enough to consider her own behavior. Even the smallest interaction had overly restrictive rules, and then she would blame poor behavior and outcome on the other person. She'd call them abusive because she had previously been made to feel unsafe in the world.

Fran's condition worsened until no one could even breathe safely around her, so tightly her rules for interaction or conversation were. So those closest to her were forced to abandon her in her time of need until she could find a way to heal *herself* enough so they could return and support her.

This is just one example of how thoughts can become so invasive and take over everything in our lives if we don't tend to them through counseling and self-healing modalities like massage and meditation while supporting the body's nutritional needs throughout this process.

People find after a really good healing session, whether it's a massage or emotional bodywork, that they are ravenously hungry and really tired. This type of work is as intense a workout as a quarterback or a linebacker practicing and getting ready for a big game or even the Superbowl. It's as strenuous as preparing for an Ironman Triathlon competition or a long marathon.

Working through emotional trauma is as taxing on the body as if you were an Olympic athlete practicing every day for the Olympics! So, if that's the case scientifically, what makes us think our body is going to be able to perform at the same level during a self-healing journey whether we use natural or synthetic means to help us without proper nutrition if a top-performing level athlete can't do it?

The body needs good nutrients.

That is our thought.

I can hear you now, saying, "Okay, okay, okay! Hold on a minute!" But in this context, applied to your own situation, aren't you too actually, performing at the same high level with your thoughts, with your stress levels, with your health situation? When we don't eat things that actually nourish us—and nourish us in the right ways (yes, it makes a difference—I give you spinach as an example—most of us have been eating it incorrectly and don't yet realize how damaging it is)—our body and mind have to work even harder to complete basic tasks, which requires even *more* of the right nutrients. You must stop and ask yourself: are you actually depleting your body of nutrients with the diet you believe to be "healthy?" *Most* people are. I was too.

Our egos would have us believe" "But not me! I'm in the 1% who eat healthy." I'm sure you are eating *some* healthy stuff. But your proportions could be off, and you might be as well be eating junk food, for all the inflammation happening in the body. "Good, healthy food can't do that...!" Can't it? Are you *sure*?

We can't base our nutritional understanding of ourselves on anyone else's requirements or expectations. Usually, our needs are more delicately balanced than we'd like to admit, but that is a trauma-ridden discussion for another day! Remember, don't let your knowledge puff you up. Tell your ego with true love, "Calm yourself down, little puffer. I'm busy learning *new knowledge* so I can walk in wisdom and light!"

Sometimes we experience a trial and nothing happens. True. Other times we eat something that's not nutritious and, again, nothing bad occurs. Sometimes it does, and sometimes it doesn't. In and of themselves, one or the other of these things don't really make that much difference.

Have you heard of epoxy? According to dictionary.com, it's a noun: also known as epoxy resin... used chiefly in adhesives, coatings, electrical insulation, solder mix, and castings. And, it's a verb: to bond (two materials) by means of an epoxy resin. It is a high strength adhesive, often made of two different materials that must be mixed just prior to use.

Epoxy usually comes with two tubes, each containing a different ingredient or chemical. You mix the two together with a stir stick and the chemical reaction between the two creates heat, which hardens the new chemical combination until the process burns itself out, and then it cools and is set. Alone, each of the two chemicals are non-reactive but once we put them together, they change and become something entirely new that they could not be by themselves.

Timing—or time—is an ingredient. Much like thoughts are an ingredient, and so is toxicity. Each separately are relatively harmless enough, but once we start mixing them all together at the same time, they heat up and create something entirely new. Even mixing *two* of these together, while not desirable, are not going to create and become what the three together will create: a chemical reaction in the body, exponentially increased!

The body tries to get out attention to address any issues at hand like a quiet, shy, polite child who walks up and whispers to you that they need a drink of water or maybe even tugs lightly at your clothes to try to tell you they're tired or hungry. As the need increases, they may begin to whimper or, if they're beyond self-control, even throw a tantrum.

These signals are so quiet that, in the rush and bustle of our culture and our noisy life's "to-do's", it can be easy to ignore, push them aside, or even rationalize that we don't *deserve* to and can't possibly take the *time* to slow down for even a minute to take care of ourselves. In fact, society rewards us for ultimate self-denial in all areas. The more self-depreciating you are, the more awesome, the more worthy, the more valuable you're told you are.

But it's a lie.

It's a lie concocted by those who wish you harm, by those who will profit from you falling into disease, by those who don't want to see you fulfill your great life purpose. Who are those people in your life? *Don't let them win.* Do what's healthy and balanced, nourish yourself, and use foods the right way in order to cleanse *and* nourish your body.

Back to time. Time is sneaky. It can disappear without your even realizing it. You can lose it. It can be wasted, squandered, made, it has super powers: it can fly, especially when you're having fun. It waits for no man or woman. It can be eaten up, it can put you out—as in *time out*—and it can pass without dying. One of the many things that has a past, present, and a future and still does not exist as we know it. It's time.

Time is so elusive and powerful. It is soft and doesn't stop to grab you. It marches on as if it had not a care in the world. And this makes it like the stirring stick for the epoxy of thoughts and toxicity: the moment these three things collide all at the same time, it starts a reaction. The difference is that epoxy's reaction is fairly quick, whereas timing, thoughts, and toxicity take a bit longer to stir together and form a reaction. This is a good thing because, if we exercise wisdom (which requires us to de-puff our present knowledge), we have time to reverse the effects before it becomes a much larger, more difficult problem to manage, *if* we address it.

Before she left it, Fran's situation had been brewing for quite some time. If I recall correctly, it had been going on for months or even years at a highly intense level, despite her repeated requests, complaints and entreaties to those who might be able to help her get the relief she required. Her situation was so bad for her, it made her weep bitterly every day while it was going on. She didn't want to leave. There was so much good surrounding the relationship, but her abuser exhibited toxic and inappropriate behavior. She finally decided to get out, which got her away from the situation, but it also caused great regret and grief for the good things she had to leave. This silently stirred her resentment unbeknownst to Fran.

Time passed, as it does, and Fran forgot all about what happened. This, coupled with her poor nutrition, the timing of the onslaught, and the toxic emotions all brewed together, unheard, and undealt with for years until the physical manifestation of her cancer seemed to pop up out of nowhere.

Once Fran started her cancer treatments, she called her friends and family for moral support and prayers on her behalf. It's smart to build a wellness support team, and it's even smarter if you get everyone all working on *their own* physical, emotional, and spiritual stuff, too, so that you can encourage each other.

Fran also called me, and we started working on adding new knowledge to increase her odds at helping her body also contribute to her healing process by learning to put it more in balance. She de-puffed her ego, learned new, better habits and is continuing with her new nutritional practice. She said that she has noticed a big difference.

The body is great at soliciting (or, asking for) our help to stay in balance. It whispers quietly, inspires us to hold self-healing points on the body that can help organs, and sometimes it will even cry and yell at us. If Fran's story can teach us anything, let's take away these ideas:

1. Pay attention to your body.
2. Take care of imbalances early.
3. Foods *do* make a difference.
4. Watch out for timing, thoughts, and toxicity.
5. Work through emotional trauma right away.
6. Don't let the ego get in your way. De-puff!

There was a group of missionary men who had gone out to teach the world about Jesus, and they had just all returned home around the same time. It was a joyous reunion for them. During this occasion, the topic came up about the signs that follow those who believe in God. I'm sure they had probably seen many mighty miracles on their journeys. One of the things they mentioned was: in Jesus' name, they would heal the sick. [6]

Fran invited her friends and family to join her in group prayers on her behalf. Armed with the knowledge of the root cause of her malady and an improved nutritional plan, she felt well-armed going in to a prayer battle.

Each time they got together and prayed over her, she said that she felt healing come into her body. Was she healed all at once in one prayer?

FRAN'S 6 TAKEAWAYS

1. Pay attention to your body.
2. Take care of imbalances early.
3. Foods *do* make a difference.
4. Watch out for timing + thoughts + toxicity.
5. Work through emotional trauma right away.
6. Don't let the ego get in your way. De-puff!

No. Not all healing happens that way. And not all causes of dis-ease or illness are so easily removed. It depends on many factors. But, eventually, she was healed completely, with a combination of her cancer treatments, improved nutrition, and prayer groups.

Fran's experience entirely changed her and helped her want to put her life more into balance—and she did. I'm so grateful for Fran and her experience! Even though she was initially resistant to considering there might have been an experience so painful that she had forgotten it, she worked up the courage and was willing to be open to new things. It changed everything for her.

One of the biggest things in life that we need to hold onto is hope. Did you know, a group of scientists did an experiment on a group of rats to see how long they could swim? Initially, they just timed the rats until they gave up and drowned. The next time, they put the rats in water and just when they were about to give up and drown (like the first time), the scientists gave the rats help by plucking them out of the water and letting them rest.

Each time, the scientists waited a little longer before helping the rats out of the water, finding that each time, the rats kept swimming longer before they actually gave up. Once they reached a certain point, the scientists decided not to help the rats anymore, and what they found was that the rats just kept swimming because they had been conditioned to know that eventually help would come, if they didn't give up. The rats kept swimming—for 60 hours! Because the rats believed they would be saved, they were able to push their bodies well beyond what the scientists had previously thought.

I don't know about you but, I think that is inspiring! Our bodies are capable of so much more than we give them credit for if we *don't give up*. And imagine what they can do with the right nutrients in them and when they are in balance. Nutrition plus hope. That's what Fran had. She had nutrition, balancing, *and* hope.

So, what is *hope* exactly? Merriam-Webster.com says that *hope* is a verb:

1. To cherish a desire with anticipation, to want something to happen or be true
2. Trust to expect with confidence, reliance

In *Strong's Concordance*, *hope* as a noun is: a gathering together a pool, abiding in.

Hope *does* eventually require some actual work and effort on our part, then. David was a king of Judah, pretty well-known and popular, who slayed a giant named Goliath and won the whole war for his nation by slinging a stone when he (David) was still a boy. King David really loved psalms. Psalms are songs, praises, prayers, and other compositions that make up the nineteenth book in the Old Testament of the Bible.

The songs, stories, and poems in the Psalms are usually based on some level of knowledge or experience that the writer had. This particular psalm references blessing God, who forgives all our iniquities (a fancy word for *sins*: everything from ignorant transgressions to full blown choosing to do evil). The psalm also mentions that God heals all diseases. [5]

Iniquities are mental choices that become physical decisions we make to break the laws of health and ultimate happiness (out of ignorance or rebelliousness), whether against ourselves or against another person. God is quite clear: we cannot stay intentionally ignorant because he still holds us accountable to search out knowledge.

Diseases range from, as mentioned before, genetic malformations and imbalances caused by exposures from chemicals to traumatic experiences, bacterial overwhelm, poor choices, spiritual maladies, and more. We cannot look upon someone and say "That man is blind because he or his parents sinned!" While that is possible, it's very unlikely, and in this world filled with poisons and malnutrition, it's more likely that other factors are at play. You have to look at *all* the factors. Unfortunately, most people are not sufficiently trained or qualified to do so, let alone, *interested* enough to look that deeply into all the factors.

It is a pretty big claim to say God heals all diseases, but it must be based on quite a bit of substantive experience. The Bible is full of examples like this. I won't take the time to go into these claims in this book because our main focus is on the importance of foods, but feel free to just go through the entire Bible researching all the diseases God heals in it. You'll be quite impressed. Start mastering the art of nutrition and see how many diseases *you* start to heal and prevent in your own body!

We've touched lightly on the fact that not having enough of or not having the right nutrition can be damaging to the body, create imbalances, and create a diseased state within the body, but what about having too much or excess?

Excess will *also* create massive imbalance in the body. "But not healthy foods, right?" Yes, even healthy foods can create imbalances. There are various things that can lead to excess consumption; things like addiction, ignorance, lack of other sources of food, etc.

When done properly, fasting can be very beneficial for helping bring the body and mind back together and help build self-control. Note, though, that it should be more than just abstaining from food and/or water for a period of time (generally twenty-four hours). Done this way, studies have found results to hardly be any different than starving the body. A *true* fast requires a voluntary abstinence from food and drink *with the purpose of developing spiritual strength.*

In the New Testament of the Bible, records show fasting was regarded as a natural way of showing sorrow. It was often combined with other ceremonies like a rending of the garments (a Jewish and Christian tradition of tearing outer clothing worn at room temperature near the neck and on the front, made in a specific way to psychologically express grief and mourning and thereby gain relief), putting on sackcloth, refraining from washing the face or anointing with oil.

But ceremonies go beyond the acts. They involve a dedication of the heart—a commitment of the mind and heart together—towards a higher, nobler purpose. Sacrifice brings blessings *and* benefits. Anything worth having is going to require some sort of sacrifice, and the same is true with our nutritional goals. Science has shown that fasting once a month for twenty-four-hours to be the most beneficial. If we want to get great results, it's going to require us to give up what we think is good for what is better. Fasting teaches us that principle and it's healthy for the body.

Regular monthly fasting not only allows the stomach and intestines a chance to have a rest period from constantly gorging ourselves with tasty vittles from sun-up to sundown (or, for some, all through the night), it also gives us a chance to slow down and reflect on other ways to improve ourselves. It allows us the opportunity to become just a little bit more self-disciplined in our lives with food *and* with our thoughts, feelings, emotions, and even behaviors.

One of the greatest accomplishments we can make in our lives is to learn to conquer ourselves. This is *the* greatest demonstration of power and control. The world has it backwards, trying to control situations and/or other people instead, which gives only a false sense of control and removes the ability or chance for each individual to master their own self.

Since this ability will vary from one person to the next as to *what* they need to learn to control, as well as how weak or strong they are starting out, they need to realize that the timetable will also look different from one person to the next. The way a person's brain works, nutrition levels to support the learning processes in the brain, the emotions of the heart, and the willingness of the body to cooperate, too, will all affect these things.

Fasting helps us focus in on our purpose. It puts our passions and appetites on hold. Like any muscle in the body, the more we use it and exercise it, the stronger it becomes. Pure, healthy foods leading up to a fast during the month will nourish the body so it can sustain itself when you abstain. We ask God to bless the efforts extended to him, and hand over our will, to be in alignment with the ones who can make transformation happen. And, we get to be part of that process. What a wonderful thing!

There was a guy named Alma who used to be a high priest for a really wicked king. Alma was young and foolish, delighting in if not enjoying (perhaps) the affluent position he held—until he had an experience that woke him up and he realized his awful lifestyle was based on a bunch of lies! The king would have had him killed for standing up to him and the other high priests when sharing his new-found realization, but Alma ran for his life and was protected in his hasty flight.

After Alma learned this new life-changing information and he was made painfully aware of the error of his ways, he began going around the nearby towns sharing with anyone that would listen. That's pretty typical human nature. You learn something new; you want everyone to know about it, right?

Some people received Alma and his message openly, and others violently opposed what he was sharing with them. After all, these ideas not only went against what they *had* believed but was also against the king's requirements of the people living in the land. One such town was called Ammonihah named after its founder.

The people in Ammonihah had hardened their hearts and would not even *listen* to Alma and what he tried to share with them. Even though Alma prayed mightily, even wrestling with God, his mighty prayer on behalf of these folks didn't make a dent in their hardness.

The people told Alma, "We know who you are, Alma, the high priest of the land, but guess what? We're not members of your church and we don't believe in your foolish ideas. Also because of that and the fact that you gave up your position as a judge, you can't even judge us! You have no power or authority over us. Get lost!" They yelled at him, spit on him, and threw him out of their city.

I'm sure you can imagine how bad Alma must have been feeling. There he was, going around and trying to right the wrongs he had helped commit against these people. He's thrown out of town, he feels depressed, and he's been fasting a long time. (*At that time, long fasts were an expected, natural way of showing sorrow.*) All this was going on when the angel of God shows up and tells him to go back to Ammonihah with a more *clear* message, and specific directions.

With renewed urgency, Alma turned back and returned to Ammonihah, but he snuck in another way since they were watching for him. At this point, he was starving because not only had he been fasting all that time, he had also been walking for some distance. In those days, a person such as Alma would have done a lot of traveling and been dependent on others for food and short-term shelter while doing their work. So, he walked up to a man and asked if he could have something to eat.

The man Alma had approached happened to have the same belief system he had, and he told Alma so. He also told him that he recognized him as being a holy prophet of God and that an *angel* had shown Alma to him in a vision and told him to take Alma into his home. So, he did. He took Alma home and fed him, telling him that he knew having him there would bring a blessing to him and to his house.

This is all to say: fasting has power. Not only physical power to bind addictions and habits. Not just to help balance certain imbalances in the body. There are also emotional and spiritual benefits as well, as we see demonstrated by Alma's story. Did you know that the name, Alma, means *"nourishing?"* He had come to spiritually nourish a people who were starving so much their spirits had become hard as stone.

Remember: the difference between fasting and starving comes down to intention, purpose, and what you've been consuming and not consuming *as well as* what's been consuming you.

It's important to note that the longer the body, mind, and heart, or spirit goes without *proper* nourishment, the more vitally *crucial* fasting becomes to regain control of the true self. The further out of balance one becomes, the less a person will *want* to fast. Why is this? It all comes down to acid/alkaline balance. Like attracts like. Maybe you've heard the phrase opposites attract. It is actually a physics impossibility and a myth that opposites attract. Doctors and physics professors all agree on this hard proven science. It is a fact that like attracts like. More acid will attract more acid. This makes the mass of *acid* even bigger. Kind of like that ol' Amalakiah who wanted to be king, running over to the dark kingdom so he could increase the size of his dark army. He dethroned the king then used the army to take over the kingdom of light and goodness and tried to make his army and kingdom even larger.

Imagine, if you will, a magnet. Each piece that gets added to it only serves to strengthen it. Out of balance, it is destructive, whether on the acid or alkaline side or positive/negative charge. The bigger it gets, the more attractive and destructive it can become. The magnet doesn't "*want*" to let go. Its *job,* is to attract *more* of itself.

Will you feed the "good guys" or the "bad guys" in your body? Who *are* the "bad guys" anyway but the ones out of balance, the ones creating too much chaos? Make a note: foods can create balance in the body, or they can create chaos in the body.

There is a really great story that exemplifies this concept in a way unrelated to food that perhaps can help you bring a new understanding to your mind. Maybe, it will even help you in the way you relate to food as well. To get a good feel for what was going on, let's step back in time a little, and let's ponder the story in relation to foods.

In this story, the land was no longer ruled by kings, but instead judges ruled in conjunction with laws of the land that were put in place by the voice of the people. As long as the people lived in balance and harmony and the judges followed and maintained the laws put in place by the people, there was peace in all the land.

However, after several generations had gone by, the chief judge died and three of his many sons decided to run for the position. This, then, split the favor of the people three different ways. One of the sons won the judgment seat by the voice of the people, and he became the judge and governor. One of the brothers who did not win, united himself with the will of the people, as he should. The other brother, also did not win, but he and the people who supported him became very angry, and he was about to rile his supporters up in a rebellion against everyone else. Right at the moment he was about to do so, he was taken and tried by the voice of the people and condemned to death.

"Whoa!" You might be thinking, "that's pretty harsh!" But the new judge's brother was not just upset he didn't get his way. The brother's *intention* was to *destroy* the *liberty* of the *people* in the entire land. The whole concept and way of living in peace and harmony—(and it worked)—was based on each and every other person being able to enjoy liberty too. The second brother *knew* this was the law of the land when he ran for office and had agreed to uphold it—until it didn't go his way.

The second brother's followers snuck in and killed the lawfully and newly elected judge and governor *(his brother!)*, and they swore to secrecy to each other never to reveal who the man was who killed the judge. Those in this murderous band of followers who were discovered were put to death. Meanwhile, the first bother (the one who had been first runner-up) was put in as judge and governor of the land, as the laws dictated.

The next year, neighboring enemies came to battle against the people of the land. Because of all the legal election troubles, the people hadn't kept their guard up around the city, mistakenly thinking, their enemies would never come inside the city to attack them because of where it was located.

Their enemies came so fast—and there were so many of them—that the people were caught completely unawares. Anyone who stood up to the enemies was killed, and the whole city was overtaken quickly and easily. Even the newly appointed judge and governor (the second one) was killed quite violently. Many people remaining in the city were put into prison. And once the enemy leader saw they had taken the strongest hold in the whole land, he became very bold and felt he could easily take over the rest of the country.

Plowing through the center of the country threw everyone off because the people had figured their enemies would attack around the outer edges along the borders of the land. The enemies had killed many men, women, and children there.

One of the generals of the land discovered the enemy's plan and sent an army to head them off. The army gave the enemy such a hard time that the enemy was forced to retreat to the capital city. Many were killed in the battle, including the enemy's leader. And, since they were surrounded on all sides without ability to retreat farther, the intruders surrendered and were allowed to peacefully leave the land.

Being without a judge and governor once again caused a lot of contention among the people. They voted and put a new man into office. What the people didn't realize was that the man who had murdered the first judge was still alive and well, and he had plans to murder this new judge too. But an expert assassin rose up and convinced this ill-intentioned group to put *him* in the judgment seat, and he would put them in positions of power and authority over the people. Does this sound familiar? But the plans were thwarted, and this band of men fled into the wilderness for fear of being caught and put to death.

For a few years, there was peace in the land (other than a few small squabbles). The population grew and spread and began to fill the land once again. Then, all the same issues began to reemerge. Things had become comfortable, but the judge and governor still ruled with justice and equity and kept all the laws. He had two sons.

Almost a decade into this tale, the wars and fighting had calmed down. The rulers of the land did not know that the band of robbers and murderers that had previously fled—now being led by the expert assassin—were still were hidden among the more settled parts of the land. Because they were hidden, they weren't destroyed.

The church grew and became very prosperous, but it was humble, and in the next decade the third judge died of old age and his oldest son took his place. The people began to fight a lot amongst themselves, and murder became commonplace. Those refusing to follow the laws of the land were driven out and went to join the town's hidden enemy. The town began warring again because of their pride and the coveting of each other's riches, and every imbalanced and evil life practice began to come about. The people lost most of their land to their enemy and eventually had to give up trying to get it back. The people of the town and land became extremely weak, and they exhibited much imbalance, chaos, and fear.

Finally, the fourth judge and governor (the oldest son of the judge who had died of old age) gave up his judgment seat to another man; the laws were made by the voice of the people and many more people had begun to choose evil over good. The people were ripe for destruction and the laws had become corrupt. Their hearts had hardened so much that they refused to obey the laws anyway unless the people were destroyed by court order.

This retiring judge had become so weary because the people had turned to evil, and he quit. He decided to go teach the people to put their lives back into balance for the rest of his days, and his brother went with him and did the same.

So, what does this have to do with food?

Actually, a lot. In the body, there is good bacteria and bad bacteria. What we eat feeds either one or the other—and not usually both. What we can learn from this story about the judges (by the way, *you* are the judge in your body), is that there is always something trying to take over and overthrow the delicate state of balance in the gut, and thus, the rest of the body.

There are things that can throw off the brain: parasites stealing food, trashing the place inside you, and taking over. These are *not* good house guests! But fasting and gaining self-control can stop the war from going on inside of us. We can cut off the supply lines feeding the enemy. We have the power to make better food choices, feed the good bacteria, clean ourselves out, and eliminate the waste by-products of this "enemy" bacteria.

Later in the story, we learn that the two men—the retired judge and his brother—not only went throughout their own land, they also went into a part of the enemy land that had once belonged to their people. There, they were thrown into prison, where they were kept for many days without food. The enemy jailors planned to kill the two brothers right there in their prison cell once the brothers were too weak to fight back.

Do you suppose the two brothers were merely languished in their cell, wasting away to nothing? Or do you think they turned their situation into a united opportunity for fasting in order to bring about miraculous results? The jailors came to kill them but dared not enter the cell because they said they saw that the brothers were filled with a light brighter than any fire.

You may not be aware of this, but the kind of foods you eat can give you a dark, gray cast or cause you to be filled with light emanating from the whole body outward. It is more subtle at times and at others highly visible. Literally: each bite you take, decides whether your body is filled with darkness or light.

Different foods burn at different temperatures and different speeds. What and *how* you eat makes all the difference. The better you eat, the more clearly you can see the change. Foods that are harmful to the human body burn too hot and are not "clean eating" foods—not the world's version of "clean eating" necessarily, but in how the foods interact in and with the body.

For people who want to be in tip-top shape and be "clean" internally, harmful foods must be eliminated almost completely and avoided at all costs. If you want the best chance in helping put your body into its balanced state, it's worth it to cut these unclean foods from your diet. Some of the foods may be especially difficult to cut out initially, but as you clean out more of the bad parasites and bad bacteria, it will become easier and easier to cut each time when you resist the temptation to consume those foods. This is the very first step: prevention!

The judge's capital city was overrun and overtaken by invaders and intruders due to naivete, general ignorance, and lack of diligence in defending the land and maintaining proper laws. Likewise, our own body, mind, and spirit can become overrun and overtaken without warning and without time to raise a defense. Often times this is when we're caught off-guard by a sudden, devastating illness out of the blue. However, things don't generally just happen out of nowhere or for no good reason.

Even a pot of stew takes time to boil.

We have been conditioned to think that to boil the stew we just turn up the heat and cook it, but stew does not simply appear for boiling without some sort of preparation and effort. First, you have to grow your produce, harvest it, wash it, and chop it up. While you chop up your produce, you warm the pan so you can begin to sauté your onions. Then, you must mince and sauté the garlic. Add the carrots in next, and then the celery, and then your soup stock and other vegetables. And *then* you have to wait...and wait... and wait some more until the heat works its way through all that liquid and food before it can even *think* about boiling. The *boiling* is the part you notice, but there's a lot that already happened before you saw anything happening at all.

If you're not watching the pot, you won't notice when it starts boiling so you can turn it down to a simmer. Or worse, you won't notice until all the liquid has boiled out and the pan burned without anything left in it! Are you running your body around and burning up your metaphorical stew and pan?

A burned pot of stew offers up no nutrients, no benefit to life. Maybe you could make soap from the ashes? No, there wouldn't be enough good things left to do anything with. How long have *you* been trying to run your body on ashes?

It's not just about eating or eating too much or too little, though that *can* be a factor. You can't just eat this right thing and *not* eat the other wrong thing, though that also influences outcomes. You must also consider nourishment: food combining, digestive typing, correct health status, and more. And that's just the physical food part of it. Another consideration is trauma: trauma around food, events you experienced while eating (or even hours later while still digesting), or even things you simply heard about during the several hours-long digestion window. This includes being nutritionally affected by the nutrients and plants nearby at the time!

Your body keeps track of the plants and other elements around you during these times and logs them as a threat too, not just the foods you've eaten or are digesting. Your brain doesn't realize which thing created the threat so it just remembers every single detail and just flags it all with a warning label in order to protect you from future threats. You're probably thinking that you have no idea what I'm talking about and that's okay. There is literally so much to understand about foods that this is why it is so vital to get professional help in relation to foods and healing.

"So, there's food, emotional and/or physical trauma or even physical injury. What else do I have to worry about?" you're thinking. "I give up already!"

No, no, don't worry. I know it seems overwhelming right now—and we'll simplify it some—but you must understand how complicated and how literally *powerful* food can be when so many voices are mistakenly saying it doesn't do anything. They don't understand the science. You aren't going to learn all this information overnight either. We not only need nourishment for the body; we also need nourishment for the spirit. And for those who are already sick, whether you presently realize it or not, you must first believe that if you take action, you can get better, you can be made well, you can be healed. Medical studies prove over and over that a person's attitude makes all the difference in getting well.

For those truly too weak to take action on healing themselves but who still believe they can recover, they should "be nourished with all tenderness," just as my husband nourished me when *I* was near death, unable to help myself. They should be nourished with appropriate "herbs and mild foods" for the conditions they have while working with any healthcare providers needed. These would be specialists like nutritionists, homeopathic doctors, osteopaths, chiropractors, surgeons or medical doctors, counselors, massage therapists, and more.

Never allow an enemy to tend to an ill person's care. Not only does an adversary *not* have the person's best interests at heart—perhaps loving the money pouring in, for example, over helping achieve a wholesome recovery—but the enemy may even go as far as intentionally poisoning the ill person, whether physically, emotionally, or spiritually. Don't accept gifts from strangers, because you don't know what might be attached to the gift – seen or unseen.

Make sure you work with people who have the same actual *belief* system as you, not necessarily the same church or religion, although they may be that too, but providers having the same belief *system.* Take care and always be discerning, night and day.

Why is this so important?

The body needs strength to let go of trauma that it has been holding onto for so long that is stored in the bones. It takes a lot of energy to remove and clear out old hormones, dead cells, and old medications that never got digested or even distributed through the body. I've seen it!

The body also needs strength and nutrients to be able to have all the resources and tools to make repairs to injuries and damage that has already been done. Even emotional bantering and cajoling can cause actual physical damage to the brain and body. Scientific studies are now confirming this as fact; it can be tracked in brain scans.

With this knowledge we must be very careful about harm created by our words (even when done unintentionally) but also with the hard and hateful things we might be tempted to say to someone else. This includes to ourselves, and our thoughts, our words and our actions. We may think we have a free back-stage pass and our actions don't have consequences, but they do.

We may cause someone irreparable harm that we cannot ever undo, all in the name of "fun" on our part. We might make the mistake of thinking "Well, I could handle that just fine, so they can too." But their experience and resource levels to handle, deal with, interpret, and recover are probably very different from yours. You don't know. You *can't* know, most of—if not all—the time. They could be on their last straw, at the end of their rope, with no resources left and no one to catch them when they fall. No energy left with which to recover. I know, because it happened to me!

What does this have to do with food, anyway? Everything!

The bad bacteria and parasites in the body are battling for our food and nutrients, trying to control us and make us do what will help and strengthen *them*. They can release hormones, imitate our emotions, and even make us

74

think we are having food cravings! They can make you feel afraid of the things that would harm *them* (but not you) or keep them in check—like vegetables—instead of taking complete control over your own body and mind. Scientists have found a direct connection between these critters and your thoughts and emotions.

Your body is a temple. A place for you to dwell. Learning these food nourishing skills not only teaches us to care for our bodies, it unlocks great potential, skills, and talents. Much like in a video game when you capture or gobble up a certain game piece or token and you unlock a new level, mastering the correct balance of foods and nutrition for your unique individual body unlocks new levels in your life experience.

Just as it is important to good health to clean your house regularly, it is vital to clean your body inside and out too. We talked a bit about cleansing the outer vessel in my second book, *"Fountain of Living Water"* if you'd like information and activities on that topic.

There are a lot of fad diets out there promising the world. Some of them *appear* to be creating the outward appearance you *think* you're looking for: losing weight or feeling better. And some of these things are *good* to want in some cases but there are a lot of people out there—even well-meaning nutritionists—who may not realize the deeper level of "what and how" food really affects the body. Even the medical industry, in general, does not believe food can change the body's chemistry despite seeing the results staring them in the face on completed lab tests.

The modern-day medical industry's education system is highly respected, and the medical industry does a lot of good—*I'm not saying they don't.* Still, you need to understand that in their education, they only provide one *single* four-hour class on nutrition out of the many years of training that is provided for medical doctors. It's no wonder, then, that medical doctors don't spend time talking with their patients about food as medicine! They should *at least* be referring people to nutritionists, homeopaths functional medicine doctors, and so on, but they don't even have enough training on nutrition to know they need to do *that.* That's not the fault of individual doctors. That's a training gap.

What we really want to know is: why is clean eating so important?

To have a greater understanding of this, we have to look back at the days of Noah and the ark from the Great

Flood. (I cover this more in detail in *"Fountain of Living Water"* which is a book on water and hydration. Suffice to say there's hard physical evidence proving it was a real ark—the only one of its kind and size dating back to Noah's day.) That being said, let's *assume* for this example that the story is all true. Granted, we don't have lots of written records available from that time period, but let's work with what we've got.

In Noah's day, there was great evil, genetic mutations, and things God considered abominable that corrupted all flesh—except for Noah and his family. Noah and his family must have lived out of town or something, grown their own food, and really known who God was, that sort of thing. We are told that our day (in which we now live) would be like the days of Noah. Just look at all the court documents being released and what whistle blowers are leaking; I'd say we have at least a *hint* of an idea what times were like then.

For those less familiar with the story, Noah took seven of each kind of clean beast and only two of the unclean ones, the male and the female. He also took birds by the sevens to keep seed alive on the earth. It flooded forty days and nights. The fountains of the deep broke open, and

Noah and his family were on the ark 150 days before the water subsided and they could finally get off the ark. After disembarking, Noah built an altar to Elohim, taking from every clean beast and clean bird, and he offered a sacred burnt offering to God. First, he gave thanks and rejoiced in his heart. [6] After all, God had spared his family. I'm sure his next thought was to ask God to never flood the earth again!

So, what's the big deal about clean animals?

A clean animal is symbolic of a blameless Savior who takes upon him the penalty for a broken contract and pays the price for the things we've done that have separated us from our Father in Heaven. As it is said, the price, or penalty, for this violation that mankind made is death, and Jesus' death restores us to life from this penalty so we can have the opportunity to make U-turns and make better choices. Also, how about this concept? We make a sacrifice when we choose to leave the unclean *bad* foods (beasts) alone in order to choose that which is better, or clean.

Just like Noah—God smelled a sweet savor when Noah offered up the sacrifice—when we eat clean, we will smell sweet or *clean* to God also. What does this have to do with anything?

Well, in the Bible, God gives a list of what to eat and not to eat. Get this: there's actual science behind it! It comes down to the temperatures in which foods break down in the body. It turns out, that all the so-called "unclean" animals burn *too hot*. It's like putting jet fuel in your car engine and trying to run it. A car doesn't need that much or that type of heat or level of explosion of power to run!

Gasoline's ignition temperature is 1135–1500°F (612.78-815.56°C) which is pretty close and consistent in range [***] and jet fuel burns between 800–2500°F (426.67-1371.11°C) [****], which is a huge difference. Just like different types of gas burn at different temperatures, foods do too; they are both kinds of fuel. Unclean animals digest *too hot,* unlike plants and animals that are considered *clean.* Here's a list if you're curious:

<u>CLEAN ANIMALS</u>: ox, sheep, goat, gazelle, hart, fallow deer, wild goat, pygarg, wild ox, chamois. All water critters with fins and scales, all clean birds – see below for which NOT to eat. All flesh used sparingly, during famine, and if ill.

<u>UNCLEAN ANIMALS</u>: Don't eat those that chew the cud or divide the cloven hoof. Camel, hare, coney (which chew the cud but don't divide the hoof). Swine and pigs (which divide the hooves but don't chew the cud)—don't eat them or even

touch their dead carcasses. Fish that don't have fins and scales. Birds such as eagle, ossifrage, osprey, glede (buzzard), kite, vulture (falcon), every type of raven, any type of owl, night hawk, cuckow (seagull), hawk, pelican, vulture, cormorant, stork, heron, hoopoe bird, bat. Winged insects and every creeping thing that flies. Anything that dies of itself—also don't feed to strangers or sell to non-locals).

Unclean foods lead to darkness and harm not just physically but also emotionally and spiritually, while eating clean leads to life and light in the body, mind, and spirit. There's a lot more science on this, but it's too much to go over in just one book, and I don't want to overwhelm anyone. But if you're curious, do some research on it. It's not going to be easy to find, so be patient in your search.

<u>CLEAN ANIMALS</u>

- Ox
- Sheep
- Goat
- Gazelle
- Hart
- Fallow deer

- Wild goat
- Pygarg
- Wild ox
- Chamois
- All water critters with fins and scales
- All clean birds
- See other chart of which NOT to eat
- All flesh used sparingly, during famine, and if/when ill

UNCLEAN ANIMALS

- Those that chew the cud or divide cloven hoof
- Camel
- Hare
- Coney (which chew the cud but don't divide the hoof)
- Swine and pigs (which divide the hooves but don't chew the cud)—don't eat them or even touch their dead carcasses
- Fish that don't have fins and scales

- Birds such as eagle, ossifrage, osprey, glede (buzzard), kite, vulture (falcon), every type of raven, any type of owl, night hawk, cuckow (seagull), hawk, pelican, vulture, cormorant, stork, heron, hoopoe bird, bat
- Winged insects
- Every creeping thing that flies
- Anything that dies of itself (—also don't feed it to strangers or sell to non-locals)

Now you're thinking about your food intake and perhaps you're wondering what else you can do to improve your health and increase your mental clarity. Paul, while in Galatia, mentions many things that are harmful and damaging to the body, mind, and spirit. One relates directly to food, and that is drunkenness. [7]

There are a lot of so-called research studies out there for and against alcoholic beverages. You can pay anyone to slant the results of any study to get whichever outcome you want to display depending on what you leave out and what you put in, based on my experience. So, many go deceived about true health benefits about a lot of things, unfortunately, if you don't know what to look for. You have to pay special attention and think of additional questions outside the box that the people doing the study may not have thought of or did not include, whether intentional or not that might affect the outcome for any study. This is how you can determine how accurate it may or may not be.

There are a lot of anti-nutrients in alcoholic beverages, (things the body does not like and cannot use) that rob the body of good resources. The body needs these resources for itself but has to use them up attempting to get rid of the anti-nutrients to minimize harm to itself. It takes energy to clean out garbage. You can imagine if you're taking in an overabundance of a food or drink with too many anti-nutrients in them how much that will deplete the body as is the case, nutritionally, with drunkenness. If your goal is to be strong, healthy, and well, then using up more resources than you're taking in won't help you.

There are other issues that can tax someone's emotional well-being such as being in a position they normally wouldn't be: experiencing rape or assault, getting in a car accident, being injured or even killed, losing money, physically fighting another person, or taking drugs that damage the organs and brain. Many of my clients have told me that they quit drinking alcohol and started noticing they felt better, could think more clearly, and could easily remember details they used to struggle to recall.

The people I talked to were not even alcoholics seeing these types of results. These were self-reporting casual social drinkers! If you're finding difficulty quitting this or any other undesired habit, look to emotional, mental, and spiritual issues as well as nutritional imbalances. You must have the nutrients and strength to hold onto the changes or they won't stick and you'll have to work on releasing trapped emotions and memory fields to give yourself the strength to make the physical changes in your diet. When you hit a plateau and feel you're not progressing, it's time to change something in order to level up, so to speak.

The National Institute on Alcohol Abuse and Alcoholism provides research-based information on drinking and its impact. [+] They found that drinking too much once or over time can take a serious toll on the body's health. These are just the *physical* effects, mind you. As the body, mind, and spirit are interconnected, there are emotional, mental, and spiritual consequences as well.

<u>BRAIN</u>: alcohol interferes with the brain's communication pathways, disrupting mood and behavior, making it harder to think clearly and move with coordination. Drinking can

cause nightmares, inability to sleep well despite feeling drowsy. The actual brain may begin to shrink; learning, remembering, and maintaining a steady body temperature, become more difficult. Physical and other abuse could occur. Plus, loved ones could suffer embarrassment, grief, and loss.

<u>HEART</u>: Alcohol creates heart damage-causing problems like cardiomyopathy, arrhythmias, stroke or ischemic heart disease, hypertension and high blood pressure. Heartaches that come with having these conditions include: daily injections, organ damaging medications, expensive surgeries and health or medical equipment, and massive stress.

<u>LIVER</u>: Drinking can lead to a variety of liver inflammations like steatosis (fatty liver), alcoholic hepatitis, steatohepatitis, fibrosis, cirrhosis, and liver cancer. Cirrhosis is also caused by eating too much grain or potatoes with meat, which increases digestive alcohols in the body.

Meat and potatoes can also contribute to cirrhosis. What? I know you're thinking it's only caused by drinking alcohol, but it's not the only thing that can do it and I wanted to mention it while we are on the liver. Don't feel too bad if you weren't aware this food combo was so harmful. I didn't know either! Think how much our diets consist of things like spaghetti noodles and meatballs, hamburgers with buns and fries, pasta salads with sausage or chicken, pizzas with meat, etc. So, what can we do?

I admit, it was a difficult switch for me to make, but I wanted to help my liver out as much as possible. I decided to just worked on one dish at a time. For my spaghetti, for example, I started serving the sauce over spiralized zucchini noodles or diced veggies if I had less energy or time. Occasionally, I have regular noodles with spaghetti sauce, but not that often anymore, and I have found that it's not much different in prep work to use veggie "noodles" instead. But I feel a *lot* better after I eat!

My husband noticed a difference in how he was feeling too.

If you start today, you'll teach and train your family in better eating habits and create healthier food traditions in your household so they don't even have to think about it. Moving forward, teach them the way to eat and how important this knowledge is to pass on to future generations so they can keep it going.

<u>PANCREAS</u>: Alcohol causes this organ to create toxic substances that can lead to acute and chronic pancreatitis, a dangerous inflammation that causes swelling and pain (which can spread) and impairs its ability to make enzymes (which help keep cancer cells in check) and hormones for proper digestion. Poor pancreas functioning can also contribute to diabetes.

<u>CANCER</u>: There is a strong scientific consensus that drinking alcohol can cause several types of cancer—alcohol is even listed as a known human carcinogen. A lot of deaths are related to this!

> Types of Cancer: head and neck cancer, including mouth cancer; pharynx and larynx cancer; esophageal, especially in those who are naturally enzyme deficient; liver cancer; breast cancer; colon cancer.

<u>IMMUNE SYSTEM</u>: drinking alcohol weakens the immune system – making your body a much easier target for disease especially pneumonia and tuberculosis, slows the body's ability to ward off infections, and can cause immune dysregulation in the liver, colon, breast, oral cavity, and rectum

<u>CARDIAC</u>: cardiac arrhythmias, cardiomyopathy, ischemic heart disease, hypertension

<u>GASTROINTESTINAL</u>: Drinking can create leaky gut, microbial dysbiosis, colorectal cancer, ulcers, gastritis, diarrhea, heartburn, frequent urination, and dehydration.

<u>NEUROLOGIC</u>: Alcohol is a significant contributing factor in ischemic stroke and hemorrhagic stroke.

<u>LUNG</u>: Drinking alcohol can cause acute respiratory distress syndrome and pneumonia.

<u>MUSCLE</u>: Drinking often creates myopathy and general wasting, including less muscle mass and overall weakness.

<u>BONES</u>: Alcohol contributes to impaired fracture repair, reduced bone density, and osteoporosis.

Drunkenness can cause seizures, dehydration, injuries, vomiting, coma, and even death. And remember: changes start within the body start within *seconds* of the first *sip* of alcohol.

It's no wonder, then, that Paul instructed Titus—a Greek he had converted to Jesus's way and sent him over to the church in Crete. In Crete, Titus was to set up bishops to help educate other of Christ's followers in the ultimate way to be healthy. Only those found to be blameless stewards were called to teach and be responsible for these teachings in their community. They could not be self-willed or, as the Greeks called it, obstinate or arrogant. These bishops were not to be quick to anger, *not wine drinkers*, and not strikers (someone who beats another person). Finally, they could not be prone to filthy lucre: bribes or coveting money or possessions. [8]

You *can't* teach what you don't know, after all, and you can't think clearly or be as effective if your body and brain are not working properly. *Wine* causes drunkenness, but it's not the only thing that does. Improperly combining food can do it, too, and it's not called "being drunk on power" for nothing... You get the idea.

So, here's a little challenge for you. If you drink alcoholic beverages a lot, start cutting back, and make sure to pay attention to how you feel over time as you do. Most likely your body may need some clean-out time, which may feel icky. If it's too much, back off and continue more slowly so it's more manageable and slowly decrease your intake. Keep track over time of how you feel physically. What do you notice emotionally? You may feel more cranky initially, during the clean-out phase. It can be helpful to get help during this process, and not just for moral support. It's always good to know what foods will best support you in feeling better faster and having an easier cleansing process too!

Work with someone like a clinical massage therapist and a counselor who can help you with releasing old emotional traumas associated with the root causes linked to the *start* of drinking alcohol—big or small—to let go of the habits and addictions behind it. This prevents likelihood of relapse and makes it easier to process everything. For example: lymphatic massage helps the body clean itself out and increases the effectiveness of counseling sessions by about 80%. (If you've gone to counseling only in the past and felt it didn't help much, that may be why.) Counseling brings up the issues, but massage helps you release the issues from the body. It's absolutely necessary!

If you only drink a little, try abstaining; see if you don't also notice beneficial results. Whether you drink alcohol or not, if you eat a lot of meat and potatoes—grains and meats together—I invite you to start with one recipe you eat frequently and find a way to adjust it so that you have meat with vegetables and salad or potatoes or grains with vegetables and salad instead. What do you notice improving as you do that?

Keep switching those one or two unhealthy food combination ingredients in your recipe as mentioned above, until almost all or most of your recipes are switched over to healthy combinations of meat with vegetables; or breads, grains, or potatoes with vegetables. Usually, the difference in taste is slight. The biggest challenge for me was nostalgia from childhood memories and wanting things to remain exactly the same. But now I don't care so much about those things because I'm creating new nostalgia. The changes don't disturb me any longer; setting and locking in these new food memories will be worth it for generations to come.

Regarding fluctuating body temperatures: there is a lot associated with this phenomenon. The level of alcohol in the bloodstream, is one part of this; infection in the body, whether the result of a weakened immune system or trapped emotions, is another. We've already discussed how drunkenness and alcohol consumption can affect body temperature and create too much heat in the body. Let's talk a little bit more about fever in relation to trapped emotion and emotionally unresolved trauma.

If you're unacquainted with the concept of emotion being the root cause of many illnesses, *Prevention Magazine* [++] stated that emotional turmoil it conservatively 90% of all psychological roots.

Michael Wickett states that the "Law of Control was an essential law in understanding how we function. Many psychologists today, if not most, have come to the conclusion that the degree of control that we feel we have is in direct proportion to the amount of mental health that we have."

Wicket shows us there are no accidents. That the Law of Cause-and-Effect states: For every effect in our lives, there is a specific cause. If we do not like the effects that we are enjoying (or *not* enjoying) in our lives, it is up to us to identify (and change!) the causes.

Everything in our life happens by *law* and not by chance!

The Law of Control and the Law of Cause and Effect are completely consistent and in harmony with each other. We can control in large part what we eat, and we can control our emotions, and thus we have much *power* over our health. More power than we realize. The goal is to get the body and mind working together in harmony and overcome dysfunction.

Various experts and gurus have done a lot of research on emotional associations and possible causes linked to various illnesses. Here are a few ideas related to the emotions causing fevers:

Inability to express feelings of anger, feelings of resistance, "burning up" about something, feeling affected by the lack of order in life, and even holding onto the past.

Have you ever felt this way… to the point of becoming ill?

Not everything is caused by emotion. Some fevers, for example are caused by a weakened immune system due to eating an imbalance of foods with the chemistry acid/alkaline. Some are caused by alcoholic beverages or consuming processed sugars and foods. Human-made toxic chemical exposures and synthetics can also be a factor. We must choose carefully.

A fever is an elevation in body temperature, a symptom, not a disease. It can, at times, indicate the presence of disease or imbalance within the body. Of course, see a doctor or healthcare provider in these cases if your fever is 102°F (38.89°C) or higher in adults or 103°F (39.44°C) or higher in children. Lower running temperatures are often helpful to the body, a defense mechanism used to destroy harmful microbes. Some situations can cause complications in people with heart problems, in early pregnancy, and with dehydration, brain injury, and general discomfort.

Now that we have a little understanding of fevers in relation to foods, emotions, and illness, let's head over to Peter's house, where his mother-in-law was sick with a fever. The Savior came by Peter's place and touched (or took hold of) Peter's mother-in-law's hand, and the fever left her. She got up, and ministered to them. [9] She must have been felt a *lot* better.

Another example is when Christ went to Cana in Galilee, where the people happily welcomed him after seeing that he turned the water into wine at a wedding. There was a nobleman there whose son in Capernaum was sick, and the nobleman heard Jesus was there. So, he sought out Jesus and begged him to come down and heal the nobleman' son, who was nearly dead. The Messiah told him to go and that his son was already healing. The man believed him and went on his way. As he was heading back home to his son, his servants met him and told him the good news. His son was alive! He asked them the time he started getting better and they told him, "Yesterday at the seventh hour the fever left him." So, the father knew it was the same time the Messiah told him his son lived. [10]

Here's a third example regarding fevers and demonstrating that not only Christ has the power to heal, but we regular mortals can as well. This story is about the apostle Paul: during his journey, he had to stop at an island called Melita. He stayed temporarily with the chief of the island, a man named Publius, who very kindly let Paul and his travel companions stay with him for three days. They learned that Publius's dad was sick in bed with a fever and what turns out was dysentery.

Basically, dysentery is an intestinal infection—a really bad one with lots of really icky symptoms in addition to fever. It's not pretty and it's a lot to unpack both medically/physically and emotionally and due to its graphic nature, I'll let you look it up if you want to know more. Suffice to say, Paul went in and laid his hands on the father and gave him a blessing, and the father was healed. [11]

These three examples have the fingerprints of different types of possible and probable causes. As you review them, what do you think they are? Physical/medical, emotional/mental, or spiritual? Do you think food choices contributed at all? As you ponder on this, you can begin to understand why healthcare providers properly trained in nutrition and healing play such an important role in our health balancing act. A person thoroughly trained in all the aspects of nutrition has just as much training and education in nutrition as a medical doctor does in medicine. There is *so* much to know. What you don't know that you don't know can hurt you and others. We give you the basics of where to start and then get additional help to really reach your specific health needs and goals.

Chapter 3
Gerald:
Mental Health

WE'RE GOING TO SWITCH GEARS a bit from a physical focus to mental health. This is a tragic tale and in order to lighten it up a bit but still get its foundational point across, let's start this story with the classic line: "Once upon a time…"

Once upon a time, there was a small, little town, and in the small town was a small, small, little boy. He was tender, he was fair, and he was as sweet as could be. He was gentle and sensitive, and he was nurtured initially under a kind hand. Unfortunately, kindness became the ignorant hand of selfishness, desperation, and cruelty. Because he was so young and naïve to life, he was not able to communicate much yet. He was still trying to learn what his feelings were and what they meant or how to share them, but I'm getting ahead of myself here.

It should be the goal of any good parent to raise a child in compassion and to show the child what conditional and unconditional love is, how to properly express that to others, and how to receive the same. We hopefully strive to do better than our own mother and father by learning from their mistakes and trying to replicate what worked well. A parent can only do as well as they, themselves, know how to do; a parent has absolutely no control over a child's interpretation or understanding of things they see, feel, and perceive but they should try to do good.

The body, mind, and heart develop in stages, in order. With the proper wisdom in place, proper guidance can be given, greater understanding applied, and better results can generally (hopefully) be expected. Some spirits, some souls, however, are naturally rebellious and want nothing to do with goodness, kindness, or love. It is what they choose.

There is a difference between choosing brokenness and being stuck in brokenness at the hand of another with no idea how to ask for help. Children, and sometimes even grown people can fear for their own safety, unable to express that something is wrong. That's right. Safety. *Some* of these things can be affected and made worse (or better) by the correct use of proper foods. And this very young boy—still a babe—had no control over any of that.

With family genetics, poor environment, and inherited toxic exposures, the boy—let's call him Gerald— had a bit of a rough start out the gate. But his parents and older siblings had no idea, thinking all was fine. Perhaps there were some rose-colored glasses involved. They lived and enjoyed every bit of life. Everything felt new and exciting, an adventure around every corner. All things went and functioned seemingly as they should. There was a perfect balance of ritual, stability, routine, and fun.

There is an expected order to things in life: you are born, you live, you learn and grow and have experiences, and then you die. That's the tidy little plan. This is not necessarily all there is to it, though, and for some that plan is very short and others very long. For most of us, it's somewhere in between. As in all things, there is also the element of surprise, life unexpected, great sorrows, sickness, and health. There is opposition.

They say no one makes it out of this life alive.

Sometimes our health, even our mental health, can take a serious turn for the worst, as was the case for Gerald. No, not *worse*. Worst. With mental disorders and emotional assaults piling up, sometimes daily, and possibly even brain damage due to the traumas he lived through, his personality flipped and changed seemingly overnight, and everyone who knew this once sweet, kind boy could attest to the 180° shift. But no one knew what to do about it.

Gerald's parents took him for a visit to a young, inexperienced counselor, still metaphorically wet behind the ears, as they say, who had hardly any conversation with

Gerald's parents, dismissed their concerns, and told them that what they thought was going on was an impossibility in a child so young. So, his incredulous parents returned home with their young charge. Because they were also young themselves and of limited resources and access, they did not opt to drive to another town for a second opinion. Instead, they unsuccessfully tried to manage his increasingly poor behavior themselves, attempting anything and everything they could think of that probably would have worked on a normal, healthy child. But Gerald was neither normal any longer nor healthy.

Let's back up for a minute. Moses is credited with writing what is known as the Book of Genesis in the Bible. The first book of his that we know of him writing was called Genesis, which means: "In the Beginning" and that is also the first line.

Many people know the first chapter of Genesis talks about the creation cycles of the heavens and the earth and all that dwelt thereon at the time of its making: the water, the day and night, the plants, animals, and the crowning achievement: man and woman.

When the first male and female were being given the grand tour of the Garden of Eden, they were told that they had been given every herb-bearing seed upon all the earth, every tree all bearing fruit and seeds, and that it was meant as food for them. [12] Not just for them, but for all the animals too! There is so much evidence documented that plants and herbs can do a great amount of good when used appropriately, not just to nourish the body, but to lighten the mind and uplift the spirit as well.

We need look no further than King Saul, the first king appointed by the prophet Samuel over the then United Kingdom of Israel, to find someone who didn't use his resources appropriately or in the right time and place. Initially, it looked like things were going really well for him as a ruler. He was a good guy, but he kept seeking his own way of doing things and making bad choices that would eventually result in the end of his kingdom.

Saul and his company were at odds with the Philistines. Saul's son, Jonathan and his armor bearer, snuck out from Saul's camp and pretended they were switching sides to join the Philistines in order to get the Philistines to drop their guard. Then, Jonathan and his armor bearer killed twenty men and ran back to Saul's camp. The Philistines went crazy with confusion, not knowing what had just hit them. Saul, not knowing what had happened but wanting to take advantage of the situation, grabbed a bunch of men to go fight the Philistines. Unfortunately, he neglected to find out what God's instructions were from the priest first, as was the tradition.

Saul became so obsessed with his own plan that he cursed anyone who ate a single bite until the evening so he could be avenged of his enemies. [13] When Saul's son Jonathan came back from his sneak attack on the Philistines, not knowing his father's order to not eat anything, he ate some honey in front of the other men. Then, he told them they should just have eaten, and why not eat all their enemy's animals they'd slaughtered and enjoy the spoils? They'd have strength and feel better. This caused the people to eat things that weren't good for them and to violate God's law, losing his favor.

For more information on this topic, you can research not eating blood, not eating animals that have died in the wild in their pooling blood, and other reasons why God would command animal destruction in certain wars. One thing is, the life of that animal is in its blood. I will not be covering this information, but it is backed by science.

For the purpose of Gerald's story, we will focus on Saul telling his men not to eat all day and how that relates to food. First, Saul was not holding a fast when he demanded no food until his enemies were killed. If you recall, going without food *without* a spiritual purpose (or for self-improvement or for the benefit of someone else) is merely starving the body, and that creates mental depravity. Saul set his men up for failure and less-than-clearheaded thinking, and when Jonathan introduced a bad but tempting suggestion, the men lost control of themselves.

Food should not be used as a punishment nor a reward. Doing so can have devastating consequences. Recall the idea of timing, thoughts, and toxicity: here we have little Gerald, who was introduced to mentally destructive experiences that he couldn't begin to understand. Due to his very young age, he was never taught good coping skills. The people around him used food as a weapon and reward to try to keep his highly inappropriate behaviors under control, and he was doomed. Though he was sent to bed without dinner and beaten by frustrated caregivers trying to gain control, Gerald acted out even more. Then, his parents would reward him with food and in other ways out of guilt for such harsh punishments, hoping it would encourage him to be good.

Inconsistencies, confusion, and a complete loss of self-control and discipline reigned, and chaos in the household and elsewhere ensued daily. This led to worse eating habits, throwing off Gerald's body's chemistry further. His mental state worsened, and he became more violent. Soon, Gerald snuck into his favorite sources of processed sugar foods any chance he could to soothe his stressed brain and to stick it to his parents. "You can't tell me what to do!"

The sugar only anchored his anger more deeply and nurtured and rewarded him to increase his violent attacks. He became mentally unhinged with his false sense of power and control while simultaneously out of control. His misconceptions about life, relationships between men and women, appropriate behaviors for children and adults were all left untreated, and he quickly fell into various addictions.

When the small percent of the Israelites left with Moses from Egypt to worship and follow God, it was much harder than they thought it was going to be. They complained about everything constantly. We can't blame them, though, because change is hardwired into the brain to feel uncomfortable—scary, even—in order to protect us.

While they were walking through the wilderness, the Bible says the Israelites ate "'angels' food: he sent them meat to the full," it says. [14] This reference is to the manna God sent the Israelites from heaven each morning. A lot of research has been done on manna. Why manna of all things? It has been found, interestingly, to be high in natural inulin, which helps increase the healthy bacteria in the gut, which allows the body to absorb and use more of the nutrients that is being eaten. When eating the wholefood source, you get a lot more out of it than taking a single supplement of it. This is important to note.

According to the Bible, manna could not be reserved or stored and had to be picked daily, which points to our daily need to rely on God to get us through each day. It may have been bland eating, but—unbeknownst to the Israelites—it was also purifying them nutritionally to become God's chosen people so they could go out to lead and teach all nations. Eating manna helped to pull them away from their acquired food addictions, mental addictions, and behavioral addictions.

After a period of being grateful for not starving, the Israelites began to complain loudly about this "angels' food." They were short-sighted and did not understand the ways of God, yearning for their old style of life, old habits, old foods: "At least in Egypt, we had meat!" they said. They wanted to go back to what they knew, what felt familiar and safe.

Like Israel, Gerald also complained loudly. He complained loudly. He complained about the food he had to eat, his home, his life, and the rules. Nothing good made him happy. And because they had complained so much, God finally sent the Israelites so much quail to eat that they gorged themselves and made themselves sick on all that meat they weren't used to eating. And likewise, Gerald's parents also gave in and gave him what he wanted, as much as their meager finances could afford, but it was never enough.

Gerald had abundance, more than he could possibly need, but he gorged himself on all the things that did not fill the empty, unmet void within his psyche. His parents were at a loss, and they threw the empty things that he wanted at him, and so the emptiness within him grew like a giant black hole sucking in everything in its path. Gerald was never satisfied and ever hungry.

The apostle James was the half-brother of Jesus (Jesus was also known in Hebrew as Yehoshua). James said something interesting on the matter of not filling the requirements of both sides of a thing. He stated that if a person were naked and destitute and someone told them to "leave, peacefully" and be warmed and filled but *didn't* give them any warm clothing so they *could* be warm, what's the point of saying it at all? And if you did not give the poor and hungry any food so their belly could be filled, what good is the advice "go and be in peace"? [15]

Such was the case with Gerald. He was emotionally and psychologically naked and destitute and being *told* to be warmed and filled and to go happily on his way without being given what he really needed to cover his broken mind and warm himself, to eat and be filled. He could not! And even when he was offered it, he would refuse to accept it. He had no emotional clothing and no psychological funds to buy what he needed, and so there was no peace. There was no peace within Gerald's mind or heart—and if he could not have it, his family would not either.

As Gerald grew, his reign of terror also grew in ferocity and violence. His appetites and addictions become all-consuming and he grew weaker and weaker to resist all that ruled over and controlled him, until he was bent out of shape 180° in the wrong direction. He became emotionally and psychologically very much like the woman in the synagogue on the sabbath who had a spirit of infirmity for eighteen years. She was bowed together and could not stand herself up straight.

Likewise, Gerald was stuck that way and could not lift himself up.

If only Christ had been in Gerald's mental synagogue and called him over like the Savior did for this woman and said "Thou art loosed from thine infirmity" or, in other words, "You are free from your illness." [16] Christ laid his hands on her "and immediately she was made straight, and glorified God." She believed he could do it, and she trusted in him to help her. She did what he asked of her to do: she was in the proper state of mind to be receptive, an open vessel. She was ready to let go of the Spirit of Infirmity. Her heart was soft. And that was the difference between this woman and Gerald. Receptivity and an open, gentle heart.

To find the proper information on true, natural nutrition, how to use it, and where to find it, you will have to seek out a highly trained nutritionist, a naturopathic doctor (not just a "green" medical naturopath), a doctor of nutrition, an osteopathic or functional medicine doctor who has spent an equal amount of time studying foods and nutrients as they have medicine. Make sure to do some research because some will be more pharmaceutically leaning. If your goal is to become someone who eats more natural foods, you will want to find the right person for you.

This is one of the first steps that Gerald's family should have taken: making sure his diet was adequate for his age and trauma to give him the strength to work through his trauma and maintain the changes along with someone who could help him address the mental brokenness he was living with inside his mind. His parents didn't know what to do because they stopped before they had a diagnosis, but I'm sure they tried their best. However, that does not excuse him as an adult, now that Gerald can take control of this situation himself. He can start healing his lifetime of emotional damage as soon as he's ready to escape his pain.

Many schools train nutritionists from a medical or pharmaceutically controlled mindset, which primarily looks at the physical body only and does not consider the emotional and spiritual sides of a soul as part of the problem and solution. In the present day, synthetics are used and sold in stores often instead of the more natural approach to healing medicine, which uses actual food and food-based dietary supplementation as a primary source of prevention and health aid.

For best results, look for someone who not only has a strong grasp of how the medical world works but also how foods interact with medications. If the nutritionist understands health issues and pathologies more than just the average provider, you'll do just fine.

Food is powerful enough to kill or to heal. Those who don't know, don't believe it. Those who do and have experienced it don't just believe it, they *know* it! I am in that camp. I have experienced it, seen it, and I know it as much as I do because I have. If and when food is used properly, the body's pH can completely change. Those who don't understand the principles of how to make it work will tell you that it's not true.

Just like a magic trick, when we first see it, we don't believe our own eyes! It goes against what is familiar and comfortable to us. We can even see the trick over and over and still think it's impossible because we are unable to figure it out. However, if the magician shows us the secret behind how the deception works, we are no longer in disbelief. We understand the working of the machine and it's no longer mysterious or vexing. It makes perfect sense, and with practice it becomes easy to us.

Nourishing the body can quickly become a complicated thing what with digestive constitutions, blood types, various muscle builds, and more. Add to that the problematic trend of food that is not-food being sold as food in our grocery stores and people and corporations who care more about making money then having a healthy community to improve or maintain their life. Then there's the harmful and dangerous things like lack of information. Even the *right* information can add up to a hospital visit or two or even a lifetime of hospital visits and stays when this information is not used in the right way or time. Can you relate? How is all this possible?

Every bite or swallow has potential to contribute to build or destroy health. It either provides nourishment for you or for parasites and bacteria (which create waste products you have to clean out, or rob us of other nutrients), creating inflammation and over-acidity or over-alkalinity, and other imbalances. Too much of either one creates imbalance and wreaks havoc in the body.

Any and all of the above possibilities can affect emotions and moods—even thoughts.

Science shows with multiple studies that all this inflammation and imbalance—even things we think—are affected and influenced by these little buggers called parasites and bacteria that run out of control in our systems. Even our own human frequencies are affected and can be received through heavy metals in our body, sent through advanced technologies influencing thought and action. This is not to say we have no choice, no responsibility, or no way out of being affected by all these possible influences. Your enemy is tricky, sneaky, and secretive, so you have to be wise, discerning, and aware.

It's important to know we need to be wise about and in regards to food. *"Fountain of Living Water"* covers the first of twelve resources: hydration. From *"Member Heal Thyself,"* we learn that being hydrated properly is the first step to a healthier life. In it, I promised to cover in more detail in *this* book about foods and how they help contribute to the hydration process. Let's get into it!

If you're not currently hydrating properly (or not sure if you are), I invite you to go back and read *"Fountain of Living Water"* and make sure that you are for best results before you continue. Perhaps even if you *believe* you are hydrating properly, I cover a lot of things you may not have associated with water and hydration that are just as important as simply drinking water that you will want to start incorporating into your daily and weekly life.

So, let's tackle the question of how food helps with hydrating the body. Have you ever tried drinking water—you're feeling so thirsty—but it seems no matter how much water you drink, it just seems to go right through you? And, maybe you even felt just as dehydrated, still thirsty, and were left wondering what in the world was going on? If you have read *"Fountain of Living Water,"* you'll recall how I discussed the need for plants and vegetation to help absorb water when there's a flood. The areas of terrain that have nothing growing there, like a barren wasteland, cannot slow down a tsunami or a deluge; neither can your improperly nourished cells. The soil, hard and cracked, is unprepared and unable to retain the moisture. It is only able to absorb the smallest amount of water. So, the water just rushes on by over the top. It needs time, and it needs prepping.

So, how *does* food help hydrate the body? First, we have to go down to a cellular level to understand this principle. Let's think of it like a little house. A well-functioning home has resources going in and refuse or waste going out. If we don't keep a home clean inside, it makes it difficult not only for the people living inside to function, it becomes next to impossible to get the benefit of the resources going in. And if you can't get resources in, it makes cleaning out the never-ending supply of trash being produced equally hard. This can cause a home to shut down. In this same scenario, cells that are not properly nourished with correct, real resources nor removal of their waste will quit working and eventually die.

The body knows the difference between real and synthetic material and prefers things that are real, clean, natural, and healthy. When we put something in it that has been altered, modified, or is fake (instead of materials it can break down to create energy for the body to function), it forces the body to use precious resources for trying to clean out and get rid of metaphorical *toxic waste*—so to speak. I intentionally used the phrase *toxic waste* for visual representation only of how concerning this problem is to the body from all perspectives combined.

If something is processed, has an extended "shelf-life," or has had to be enriched, you should take that as your first clue not to buy it, eat it, nor use or probably even touch it. Okay, I may be exaggerating slightly, but seriously: anything along those lines has had everything stripped away that was worth consuming and been replaced with fake nutrition. Do you know what happens when all the good stuff—things that nourish, protect us, and serve a good purpose is stripped away?

This is when invaders break in and take over. Bacteria, disease, parasites all run rampant and unchecked—unless you start following the laws of health right away! If we don't and continue down that dark path, shame comes upon us much like Moses when God appeared to him in the burning bush. Moses was so demoralized at that point in his life he couldn't even look at God, he was too afraid! [22] Much like deficient and dwindling good bacteria and nutrients becoming scarce and depleted, good health will cower, dwindle and die unless we are willing to fight for it, or all can and will be lost.

Did you know that leprosy actually consists of several categories of diseases including a disease sometimes found to be infectious and contagious? So, for someone like Moses to be shown by God at the burning bush how to put his hand into his bosom and pull it out showing it to be leprous, even as white as snow, and then turn it back to normal, that would be quite a feat and an impressive demonstration of God's healing power! [17]

Back then, the term *leprosy*, however, was not just used for what we commonly think of. It was also used for things like clothing and walls. Surprised? I was! These *things* were said to be leprous when they had patches of mildew or some fungus growth, like if you left your laundry sitting in the washing machine too long on a warm day or perhaps you didn't quite let it dry long enough, leaving it with that horrible moldy smell. Has that ever happened to you?

Have you ever had a foot or nail fungus? Have you had mildew or mold in your bathroom or inside the walls of your house, in a basement, or under the floors? These

118

are all indications of an imbalance of one thing or another whether caused by too much of something or not enough of the other in the environment. These perhaps might be things relating to nutrition in anything from the condition of the soil, the water, or the air to dryness, cleanliness, or other things—even emotions. It's a sign that things must be put into balance immediately if you desire to return to and maintain good health.

Naaman was a mighty man from Syria. He was the captain of the king's hosts, was considered to be a great and honorable man by his master. Through Naaman, God had delivered Syria. He was known for his mighty valor. He was very courageous; a powerful man in the world. Oh, yeah, —and he was a leper (had developed leprosy). [18]

His wife had a servant girl who had been kidnapped from Israel and kept as a captive. This young girl mentioned that if they lived in Samaria, the prophet could cure him of leprosy. Now, we don't know the exact nature of Naaman's leprosy but after having his wife's servant mention this *someone* made their way over and mentioned it to him while he was with the king. The king told him to go over there and he would write a letter to the king of

Israel and let them know Naaman was coming to see the prophet to be cured of his leprosy.

Naaman took a bunch of silver and gold and ten outfits with him to give as gifts and payment for services rendered. But when the king of Israel read the letter, he got scared that the Syrian king was trying to create a reason to start a fight with him. Sending a man to be cured of leprosy (which no one in the land really knew how to cure) would inevitably create a problem. But the prophet Elisha heard about the king's grief and he asked him why he was so worried and renting (tearing) his clothes? "Let him come now to me and he will know that there is a prophet in Israel." So Naaman went to Elisha's door. Elisha sent out a servant to tell Naaman to go down and wash in the dirty Jordan river seven times and then his flesh would return to him and he would be clean.

The fact that Elisha didn't even bother to tell him in person made Naaman very angry, and he left saying, "I thought, he would come out to me, and stand, and call on the name of the Lord his God, and strike his hand over the place, and recover the leper." He was also insulted that he was told to wash in the muddy river when there were others nearby that were cleaner in appearance.

His servants came to him asking him if the prophet had asked him to do some great thing, wouldn't he have done it? How much easier is it that he said to go here and be clean? So, they talked him into trying it, and after dipping himself in the river seven times, his flesh came again like the flesh of a little child and he was clean.

Naaman was grateful and wanted to pay the prophet Elisha, but the prophet declined any offer of payment—not just declined, but swore an oath to God he would receive none of it. Even upon being urged to take the payment, he flat out refused. Did Elisha know something about Naaman's condition or of the condition of the gifts more than that it was general leprosy? I think so.

Elisha's servant, Gehazi was not wise and a little bit greedy. He chased down Naaman and lied saying that Elisha had sent him to ask for two changes of clothing and some money to feed two visitors who had just arrived. Naaman gladly shared the items with Gehazi. As Gehazi returned, Elisha asked him where he went. Gehazi said "Nowhere," but Elisha discerned it and saw what he had done. The prophet told him that *this* was not the *time* to receive money, clothing, or anything else. He told Gehazi that Naaman's leprosy would cling to him and his descendants forever and threw him out.

Gehazi apparently contracted leprosy from contact with Naaman's garments. Elisha had *no choice* but to throw Gehazi out, or he could become contaminated too! There may possibly have been something else going on with Gehazi's overall health that made him more susceptible to the leprosy or even other factors undisclosed; we just don't know.

Foods that are "shelf stable" with added preservatives make any real life left long since gone. We can imagine Gehazi's greedy and self-indulgent nature probably carried over into other areas of his life where his goodness and wisdom were out of balance and also that his food choices reflected this. We don't know for sure, of course, but it's an interesting possibility to consider. What else might it be? Try to come up with two more reasons on your own.

The closer to living food we get, the closer we get to life force, which is what we need to create and maintain life within the body. There are lots of different food-like products and "dead" foods to buy out there that are not actually food. There seems to be more *fake* food than real at stores anymore. This where we need to learn to be wise.

There's a difference between knowing something and having true wisdom. The first relates to having seen or heard information. The second has taken, learned more, and then applied experience in relation to the data and knows when to use *OR* not use *correctly* the knowledge that's received. It's like the difference between merely hearing a thing and taking a masterclass with an experiential portion where you get to actually do and practice the thing. WOW! That's a big difference.

NOTE: You don't have to physically *do* something to gain wisdom. You *can* watch someone else and gain wisdom just as much as you can do a thing and still be unwise in that area.

Maybe you're thinking, "I can't afford a masterclass or take the time, or there's too much to learn!" It's easy to just feel so overwhelmed it's easier to shut down and do nothing. Have hope, my friend! Consider this book a sort of beginner's primer into the Importance of Foods: the second of the twelve resources covered in *"Member Heal Thyself."* We will go more in depth on that topic in this book.

If this is already overwhelming, take a break, go back and read my first book, which is going to start out with baby steps. It's just a few pages you can start with to help you get more comfortable with the idea on how and where to start. Then, come back and pick this up again later. Maybe I'll even have a master level class on foods to go even more in depth with you if you desire more knowledge, wisdom, and experience.

Let's start first with the concept of the word *health*. In Old English, this word ("hælþ") denoted healing power, deliverance, and salvation. In Isaiah 58:8 it means *healing*. In Psalms 67:2 it means *saving health,* or salvation. And in Acts 27:34, health equals, of all things, *safety*.

I know, some of you are thinking "What! Scriptures? I don't want to deal with that." And that's okay. We're just talking about definitions and originations of things. Stick with me here for a few comparisons; it will be worth your time. This is one side of the wellness triangle; take what works for you, give it an unbiased, honest chance, see what you learn and toss the rest. This book is being written to cover and help a lot of people across many different belief systems and faiths. Not everyone is going to like everything in here all the time. And that's okay. It doesn't mean it can't work for you.

I'm going to bypass definitions by the medical industry and other world or local organizations because nutrition—*true* nutrition—is not within their wheelhouse. The world of foods, nutrition, and other important aspects of health are not within their scopes of practice at all.

Merriam-Webster Dictionary gives this definition for *health*:

1. Health:
   a. The condition of being sound in body, mind, or spirit especially; freedom from physical disease or pain
   b. The general condition of the body
2. Health:
   a. A condition in which someone or something is thriving or doing well

Dictionary.com includes other words for *health*: vigor, vitality, strength, fitness, stamina – whole. The latter dictionary also references "soundness and vigor of body and mind; freedom from disease or ailment."

There are other dictionaries with more of the same, but do you know what all these lack, as nice and sterile as these different definitions are? They are like processed bread. All fluff but no real substance. They lack the *how*. What is the mechanism for how this all takes place? Let me take you back up to the Isaiah 58:8 reference once more and show you a little something you might have missed.

A lot of us have heard about the many translations and lost information of the Bible, and some may be of the mindset that the Bible is fiction. No matter which camp you are currently in, let me ask: can we not learn morals, values, and lessons from a true story as well as from a fairytale? The answer is absolutely yes! With that in mind, let's take a look at some of the specific details of this particular verse of Isaiah.

In case you haven't figured this out yet, I *love* the meanings and origins of words! Words have *power*. And they give us understanding and knowledge. In the King James Version, the most widely used version, Isaiah 58:8 reads:

"Then shall thy light break forth as the morning and thine health shall spring forth speedily: and thy righteousness shall go before thee; the glory of the Lord shall be thy rereward."

Rereward means rear guard. He's got our back. One of my favorite resources to look up original text meanings is a book called *Strong's Concordance,* also known as the *Exhaustive Concordance of the Bible.* It was constructed back in 1890 under the direction of a professor of exegetical theology named James Strong. It's a stand-alone book that includes every single word in the Bible; even "the" and "in" are listed. It also includes all possibilities of the original Hebrew (shown below as H and a number) meanings and usages for each word.

It was a monumental and monstrous project to take on, and *exhaustive* is literally the most perfect description of its contents. I will be referencing this in regard to some insights on the Isaiah 58:8 verse and I suggest that if you really want to better understand what the Bible is saying, grab yourself a copy of *Strong's Concordance* for your home library. It's a book you will love.

This one verse has twelve different *Strong's Concordance* references:

> Then shall thy light H216
> break forth H1234

as the morning H7837

and thine health H724

shall spring forth H6779

speedily H4120

and thy righteousness H6664

shall go H6779

before H6440

thee; the glory H3519

of the Lord H3068

shall be the rereward H622

When I see this, I get excited because it tells me that there is a massive opportunity to pull out some interesting concepts to consider, to take apart and examine. There's possibly even some great hidden wisdom we are not going to find in the secular dictionaries.

For a little context here, the 58th chapter of Isaiah is talking about the observances of fasting. Fasting is where you go without food or water for two complete meals of a 24-hour period, depending on the fast, but it may be longer, too.

Science has shown the benefits of fasting for rebalancing the digestive system and more, but nothing as much as when done with a spiritual goal/purpose attached to it. When done with specific focus or dedication and intent, we see more: the benefits of Isaiah 58:8.

Going back to *light* in the first phrase, just above, in verse 6 it says the purpose of a fast is "to loose the bands of wickedness." That sounds very churchy at first blush, so let's break down the words into more modern verbiage. When it says "loose the bands of wickedness" what it is referencing is putting off or breaking forth from the bonds or grief being caused by things that are morally wrong: guilt, violence, or crime that is against civil law, enemies, and unethical relations.

The goal of this kind of fasting is to undo the heavy burdens and let those whose health is being crushed or broken to go free, to be free from the bondage and slavery to foods and those who would use them as a weapon against us. We know that things like processed sugar, malt, MSG, and etc. are addicting in nature. Addiction is a type of slavery. Bad eating habits are also a type of slavery. And if this is the goal—to break free from sickness and disease so we can be healthy, happy, and strong—wow! What a loving act.

If sickness is visible in the body's *light* field as darkness and addiction that bind up our health and vitality, imprisoning it, then breaking it allows our light—our essence—to burst forth as the morning.

Have you ever been up to see the sun rise? There's this period where you can feel and sense something is building. It's about to happen, even though you cannot yet begin to see or even *imagine* how big, bold, and spectacular that moment will be when the sun first bursts over the horizon! Before it happens, you may feel like a whole lot of nothing is going on, but just because you can't see it, doesn't mean nothing is happening.

Health in this verse is referring to returning or restoring soundness. *Soundness* is "freedom from injury, damage, defect, disease, etc." according to Dictionary.com. Merriam-Webster's definition of "*soundness* as in reliability" is "the ability to withstand force or stress without being distorted, dislodged, or damaged."

As you think about the many and diverse ways a person's health can be ignorantly or intentionally harmed, how important would it be to you to have that kind of reliability and strength in your own body? You'd want that kind of knowledge, right?

The root origins for the phrase *springing forth* are "to grow, to bud, to spring forth." Did you know that a brand-new babe and a new sprout both have the densest concentration of life nutrients and resources available within them? It's not just an average amount. It is all that is needed for the task of growth: an abundance, a thickness. We're not talking fat here; we're talking a full wellness warehouse of *life* within the body.

The fact that the health will come forth *speedily* is just what you think, but *righteousness* has sometimes been misconstrued and twisted to mean dark things. It actually refers to things that are beautifully just, things of justice or what is right, just, or normal, ethical, right in speech, vindication, justification, equity, and prosperity. These things will go before you and be in front of your face.

Glory refers to honor, abundance, dignity, reputation. Rereward is to gather a collective, an individual into a company of others, to bring up the rear, to gather and take away, remove, withdraw. To be gathered to one's healthy, loving fathers and as a "rear guard", rearward.

You've undoubtedly seen people who seem literally filled with light. They have a healthy glow, a white light to their countenance—their face. Perhaps it's so bright you almost have to look away. You can have this too. It begins with fully understanding how to use water and hydration and continues next with foods.

Here's something I find interesting that the apostle Paul said about food and the traditions of the world in regards to healthy eating habits in his letter to the people at Colossae (Colosia). There were a lot of philosophical ideas spreading at the time and he warned the people there not to be fooled by those who would cheat them through philosophy and empty deceptions going against God's way to eat healthy. These philosophical ideas made people feel like they were more righteous than others for following them, but it was all based on false information.

Paul wrote to the people of the city Colossae, which was a city that placed high value on mountains and water. It had twin peaks and a river flowing through it. You can imagine the abundance of food they had growing there in this area, known today as Turkey. Many authors have mentioned this city in their writings, including Paul.

In this beautiful oasis-like setting, there had been a few complaints among the people of God's church because the people in town saying contrary things to the church about their choices of food and drink. So, Paul told the

132

church members not to allow anyone to judge them in eating or drinking (not referring to getting drunk, of course) at their holy festivals. The townsfolk had come right out and were condemning them for their joyous events, their holy days, their sacred new moons, and their sabbath days. Paul told the church that they should only listen to what God said about it and only be judged by God on the matter. They should look to him and the church members as a body who knew and understood the way things *should* go as to proper instruction in these matters.

The reason this matter—only heeding God and the church's counsel on the foods and drinks they were consuming—was so important was because it was and is vitally crucial for the people of God's church, those who follow him (disciples), to be healthy and strong. This is not expired nor outdated information. In fact, it may be more vital now than it *ever* has been.

We don't have the full information on this, as of the time of this writing, but what we are now learning about how to apply eating healthy is merely a shadow (a type) in anticipation of things that are to come. To really appreciate what this means, we must take a closer look at the word *shadow*. It's one of those words that's so easy to discuss without a second thought because we think we already know everything we need to know about it. But do we?

We know the first, most obvious definition of *shadow*: the dark figure or shape cast on a surface by a body intercepting or blocking the rays from a source of light whether resulting in partial or full obscurity. However, the definition that I believe applies most here is that of a small degree or portion: a trace, shelter from observation; an imperfect and faint representation.

Many things have been lost over time about how to hold and perform these holy festivals—even their true, full, deeper meaning. We don't know why these holy festivals and events should be done and held the way they're supposed to be done. If we really knew, we'd probably be impressed and perhaps a bit undone by the new portion we shall one day receive. But imagine, if you will, how shocked or horrified we might be if we don't even *try* to apply the little bit of knowledge that we *do* have access to today in regard to food, nutrition, and how to eat well.

When we follow the laws of something, there is a reward or some kind of consequence. In his letter, Paul tells the people of the church to make sure they don't let anyone beguile or trick them into giving up their reward for following a good law. He explains that the townsfolk just don't understand, hadn't seen, and don't know the mind of God and his higher ways. The townsfolk were puffed up in their minds with their worldly knowledge. God is the head of the church and he know all things, the better things, and the better ways, like how the body, the joints and the bands and ligaments get nourishment administered to them. He knows how they are knit together and how nourishment increases as you increase God's presence in your life.

Paul tells the people of God's church not to allow anyone to judge them in eating or drinking at their holy feasts and festivals. They should only listen to and be judged by God and look to him and to his church body for proper instruction in these things. [19] If it was important enough back then for the people of God's church to be healthy and strong, it definitely applies to us today.

This brings us back to being *wise* about our foods. Now that we understand the concept of keeping our cellular houses running clean and smooth and what outward physical appearance would and should look like, let's talk about what we need to look for. We need to consume our foods as close to them being off the mother plant as possible and after they have had a chance to fully ripen *on* the plant before it's picked. There are only a very few exceptions to this rule.

Let me preface this statement by telling you: I grew up in a farming community, and I was paying attention. This is personal knowledge. Most produce you buy at the local grocery store has been kept in a storage silo for 1–3 years before it ever makes it to the store. There are ways to accomplish this without too much spoilage. Ask a farmer. Then add to that however long it's been sitting on the shelves before you buy it. During that time those fruits and veggies are slowly dying (even with these preservation techniques), using up their own nutrients to try to stay alive. By the time you purchase it at the store, there's almost nothing left in it of much nutritional value. What can you do?

The store owner is going to keep buying unripe produce from the same commercial farms, many of which are not rotating their crops to put nutrients back into the soil, resulting in weaker, less nutritious plants. They're not letting their land have an alternating period of rest, which it needs, leaving them with depleted soils and you with wimpier fruits and vegetables.

The body does _not_ like synthetics. It does _not_ do well with pesticides, no matter how "safe" they may claim to be. The best thing you can do to offset this is to grow as much of your own produce as you possibly can and buy 100% organic heirloom from local growers who practice ethical and sustainable growing practices. Petition for healthier growing laws against bad farming. Instead of fining the good farmers for doing the right things, fine the bad farmers growing things that harm and kill. Punish them for it enough that they quit doing it. The best part you can play is to try to grow your own produce and animals to the extent that you can so that you know what is actually going into what you are consuming.

Shop local farmer's markets where you can and buy, grow, and eat local. The best of these is to grow your own so you know what is actually going into those plants. If you don't have a yard, you can still grow potted plants. The harvest from even one or two of these plants will even be better financially for you than buying everything from the store.

If you're more urban, many cities now offer local shared community garden co-op spaces. If your town doesn't have one yet, consider being the one who suggests it, and learn how to get your city involved in putting one together. There's got to be *someone* in your town who's good at growing things who'd be happy to help too, and if not, why not you! Learn and then do. Think of the accolades and praise and how many others you will help! Putting together a community garden not only will benefit you, it will help your neighbors, *and* gardening has also been shown to be good for mental health.

Depending on your local climate, you may want to start with herbs or some easy-to-grow fruits and vegetables like these.

8 Easy-to-Grow Vegetables:

1. Beans, bush or runner pole

2. Chard

3. Cucumbers (don't like them? Pickle them!)

4. Radishes (very fast growing)

5. Carrots (require sandy soil, add if needed)

6. Lettuces

7. Squashes

8. Basil (the easiest herb)

Not only are these plants easy to grow, it is very rewarding watching them go through their life process from planting to harvesting! Gardening is a great activity to get children involved in, as well, and teaching *them* will help you learn how to become a gardener.

Want an easy, low effort way to garden? I recommend the Mittleider Method. (I'm not getting paid to tell you about it, I just love it that much!) Get higher yield in a smaller, denser space with less weeding and possibly even self-watering! Dr. Jacob R. Mittleider's method uses less water and can make everything about the process feel so much easier and doable, taking only a few minutes to maintain, comparatively, once it's set up. If gardening has seemed overwhelming in the past, then try it. No matter where you live in the world he has special tips for your area, even the super-hot, dry desert of Arizona! Disabled? There are ideas for you too.

What else can you do to be wise? Timothy, the metaphorical son of the apostle Paul, got a letter from Paul talking about the time *we* live in today. In it he warned that there would be a great falling away from truth. One of the handful of things he mentions is that there will be those telling others to abstain from foods that God created to be received in thanksgiving. I can't *tell* you how many online videos and social media ads I've seen of people telling you things like "don't eat bananas, they're bad," or carrots, or eggs, or ______ fill in the blank! Remember Paul's advice in Colossians a few pages back: only let God and the church body actually tell you how to use foods, not the world and its false philosophies.

Other food-wise things you can do are more difficult if you insist on buying store-purchased products. If you have people using contaminated foods to make less-than-wholesome products—things that *used* to have a good reputation for being "natural" and healthy—and you didn't ever hear or know about the changes in those foods you thought were good, how would you know? You wouldn't and you'd be eating it unsuspecting, but it is going on.

The farther the original food gets away from you, the less safe it may be, the less energy it will be able to provide you, and the lower the nutrients it has. Grow your own produce, raise goats and chickens, and collaborate with neighbors and family members. Don't know your neighbors? This is a great way and time to start!

Learn skilled trades to have a variety of ways to meet everyone's needs, especially your own. Those who do well, especially in difficult times, are those who have four or more very different skills. One skill or resource is not always going to be needed or wanted. Or maybe someone else has already been established in that one thing. If you diversify, you have greater ability to meet your needs.

It's the same with the foods we eat. The greater the variety, the more likely the body will have a wider choice of options to meet its goals. It will also be the same with what you grow in your garden and how you rotate what you're planting in the soil. Alternate plants each growing cycle; that will in turn nourish the microbes in the dirt for the next planting of a different crop, as we discussed before.

Soil micro-organisms need variety in their diets just like we do, and since plants eat the microorganisms in the soil, they need variety too. Isaiah writes about neediness in his record. As confusing as everyone thinks his writings are, they seem to be making more and more sense to me for the times we are living in now. He's writing to God in regard to upcoming global calamities. He says:

"For thou hast been a strength to the poor, a strength to the needy in distress, a refuge from the storm, a shadow from the heat, when the blast of the terrible ones is as a storm against the wall." [20]

How can you be these things if you are not healthy and prepared to help others yourself? Our collective goal should be to be strong enough to help others, *not* be the one sitting back thinking he'll enjoy the spoils of others hard labor.

Eating right can be to our starving cells what Isaiah is saying God is to the poor and the needy in distress: a refuge and a shadow. How do people become weakened enough, to become poor? Where do the needy in distress come from? We must be on the lookout so we know what to do to prevent this from happening to us as much as possible and help each other out. A city is only as strong as its weakest link, and the body is only as strong as its weakest cell.

There is a story of a priest who noticed that the members of God's church had become wicked and their bad examples were leading those who did not believe in God on from one iniquity to another. This was bringing on the destruction of the people.

This is like our bodies. When something goes amiss, it causes more problems elsewhere until the whole body is in trouble. The priest said he saw a great inequality among the people. Some were lifting themselves up with their pride and despising others. People were turning their backs on the needy and the naked, those who were hungry and thirsty. They didn't help the sick or those otherwise afflicted.

I'm in some health issue support groups on social media, and I'll tell you what: there is a lot of suffering, need, and death just in that one area. Don't get me wrong, here: there's a lot of loving support and service, the sort you can do online as far as that goes, but for the example of cancer, let me compare to poor nutritional health. Not all cancer is caused by poor nutrition. More often it is a contributing factor, affects prevention and recovery in some cases—and rushing towards death in others.

A cancer-riddled body is quite ill and imbalanced indeed. There is a great missing need whether is it physical, emotional, spiritual, or even environmental. The aforementioned priest had a man join him years later to try to help the people in his church turn their lives back around. This second man was kind of a missionary, and the two men told the people they needed to 'make a change.'

This missionary gave the people a list of how to make the needed changes so their lives could be better and happier; but he left them with this very powerful teaching that relates this same principle to our body and foods. I'll paraphrase what he said:

"Don't think this is all. After you've done these things [the list] none of it will benefit or help you if you turn away the need or the naked, neglect the sick and afflicted or fail to impart of your substance if you have it to those in need. It'll be a waste and all for nothing."

It's the same for all that other good stuff— going to counseling, doing your hair and looking presentable, getting massages, stretching, working out, balancing your finances, living in a fine house—those things that you do on the outside. It all means nothing if your body, mind, and spirit doesn't have the supporting nutrition on the inside. Without good foods, your hair will thin and fall out, no amount of makeup will cover the dark cast to your soul, muscles become stringy and tight or solidly *hard*. Money can't buy health and you can't enjoy a house you're too sick to walk around in, clean, or decorate! It's the little things that eventually add up to the big health issues like cancer or a heart attack out of nowhere.

There's no donating to the poor and needy and then taking it back again. That would be horrible! You can't do that to a person, and you shouldn't do it to yourself either.

144

Once you consecrate yourself to wholeness, be all in or else your body is going to eventually chuck you out the door.

This information is not just for you. I cannot stress enough the importance of the role you play in the benefiting the lives of others around you with food and proper nutrition information and offering help and aid to them. You *must* visit the poor and needy and administer to their relief. Who are they? Who do you not like? Yes, I said it. Do they seem angry? Sad all the time? Disturbed? That's a sign of a huge aching need. Look for who has an obvious need. Then start there, but don't *stop* there, keep going.

There is a great definition found in the *American Heritage Dictionary*, 5th edition. It's for the word *administer*, since we're talking about doing it so much. Let's dig into what it is so we have a full understanding of the meaning.

ADMINISTER:

1. To have charge of
2. To give or apply in a formal way
3. To apply as a remedy

Administration must be done by each and every one of us so that the poor and the needy may be kept until all things may be done according to God's good law. If we want to make it out of this messy world, we must stand together unified in this cause and help one another.

Think of it like composting. When you alternate planting compost and adding other mulch to restore the soil, you end up with healthier garden harvests and ultimately healthier food. When we take the people who are struggling in these ways and nurture them, they become stronger and then, in turn, return strength to others. This results in greater strength overall. Strengthening each other strengthens the community and the land.

The more we practice healthy eating and administering to the poor and needy (having poor and needy people in your community is a symptom of the entire system being out of balance), the more we become aware of these patterns in our lives, and soon our experience becomes wisdom. We must know how, when, and where to apply the knowledge that we've been practicing—and when *not* to do things. The right time and place matters. Just like romantic feelings can be a false substitute for true feelings of love, the same can be true for health. Fake things can lead to death of one sort or another. It may or may not be literal, it may be figurative—and sometimes it can lead to both.

Earlier I mentioned being wise, discerning, and aware in regard to our foods and what we consume. If we are to know how next, to discern truth, we must first know what truth is. According to Dictionary.com, the word *discern* is a verb, an action, and it means "to detect with the eyes or with senses other than vision." It can even be a feeling or a sense of knowing something, like when you meet someone for the first time and outwardly everything looks fine, but you have this nagging feeling like something isn't quite right. Listen to your gut because *it* is *discerning*—giving information to you that you can't see with your eyes. That sense will seldom be wrong, unless you're just really bad at discerning. In that case, you need to practice more and get your life more aligned with God.

Discern means to recognize or identify as separate or distinct: like when you notice someone with an obvious handicap appears different from others around them or a rose growing in a field of daisies. Sometimes differences are not so obvious, but as we practice, we can be more skilled at telling subtle differences apart.

Another definition of *discern* is "to know or mentally recognize a thing or to see or understand the difference." Some things will be obvious, like the examples above.

Others will be more subtle and can at times be more deadly or harmful if you're not in the practice of telling the two apart, like the difference between real food and synthetic, natural and artificial foods containing things we shouldn't be eating.

I love this example written by David L. Katz, in O, *The Oprah Magazine* in August 2008. He said:

"A careful analysis of the "Nutrition Facts" panels might provide some guidance, but you would have to do a lot of math before you could discern the best choice."

I whole heartedly agree, and I don't know about you, but I don't have time for all that kind of math! The King James Version of the Bible defines the word *discern* as "to examine, prove or test; scrutinize."

The world's dictionaries sound like you can be a bit more passive about the process, but the Biblical definition indeed requires us to be—shall we say—anxiously engaged in a good cause. If we look a bit deeper in the International Standard Encyclopedia (internationalstandardbible.com), it reveals five distinct translations of Hebrew versions of the word *discern* as so:

di—zurn

(https://www.internationalstandardbible.com/D/discern.html):

> *bin*: "observe," as in "I discerned among the youths." (Prov 7:7)

> *yadha`*: discriminating knowledge as in "a wise man's heart discerns time and judgment (Eccles 8:5)

> *nakhar*: "He discerned him not, because of his hands... (Gen. 27:23)

> *ra'ah*: "Then shall ye return and discern between the righteous and the wicked" (Malachia 3:18)

> *shama`*: "So is my Lord the King to discern good," (2 Samuel 14:17)

"In the New Testament the words *anakrino*, *diakrino*, and *dokimnizo* are translated this way expressing close and distinct acquaintance with or a critical knowledge of things." The primitive root of *shama`* means to hear intelligently (often with implication of attention, obedience, etc., causatively, to tell, etc.): attentively, call (gather) together, carefully, certainly, consent, consider, be content, declare. Diligently discern, give ear, (cause to, let, make to) hear (hearken, tell): heed, listen. Regard, report, shew forth, witness.

These words have power and strength in them, and by exercising them in this way they will give *us* power and strength, much like composting for the soil and much like caring for the poor and needy for the community. How do we do this? We must research and study, actively digging for information more thoroughly than perhaps many of us would feel comfortable being satisfied with searching. It's easy not to care. Easy to not want to try. Or how about that "it's simply less work to do nothing"? In my previous books, I mentioned that work is beneficial for mankind. Not for anyone else but just for our own selves *personally*.

If you do everything for people who are capable of doing things themselves—that is, not in reference to the poor and needy who *do* need our help, but those who are able-bodied—you create weakness in them, a kind of sickness. However, it's important not to jump to conclusions that a person who *looks* healthy or beautiful or seems talented or appears capable does not need help just as much as those who look like they do. This misconception can result in deadly consequences for the person needing help due to our own lack of action and offering to help.

I've worked with *so* many clients who have been in this very boat themselves. They had a life-threatening illness but because they "looked healthy" to someone on the outside looking in, they were shunned, ignored, even told they were crazy or that it was all in their heads. This kind of rush to judgment can be the most detrimental. Some injuries cannot be seen with the eyes but are just as dangerous as (and oftentimes more worrisome than) the things you can see. It is a true test of our humanity and kindness to help and serve those who are poor and needy, especially those who do not so appear so at first glance. Sometimes we rush to help those who look handicapped who don't actually want or need help try to force our assistance on them: another thing to be careful of. It all requires discernment and true compassion.

Did you know the word *exodus* means 'a departure' in the Greek root origin? I love that meaning, and in the book called Exodus, 23:25, the Bible is speaking in relation to the Jewish celebrations. It states, "And ye shall serve the Lord your God, and he shall bless thy bread and thy water; and I will take sickness away from the midst of thee." This requires in and of itself 'a departure' away from the artificial things of the world in order to serve God, the things that: do not fill up, do not satisfy, and do not nourish.

Likewise, must partake of the foods that will give us all that God has promised us. When we apply the proper laws, the mechanisms become the key to good health. Now this was *not* store-bought bread! The grain back then was handled completely differently than it is today, creating different health results entirely. There were conditions that went along with these laws and affect how we may digest information, feelings, and experiences. Exodus 23 and Leviticus 23 tell us what must be done:

1. Keep the Feast of Unleavened Bread, the Feast of Harvest, and the Feast of Ingathering
2. Do not slander anyone by false report or be a false witness
3. Do not go along with the mob mentality doing evil
4. Do not subverting justice
5. Help your neighbors
6. Stay far away from false accusations and charges
7. Don't murder the innocent or righteous
8. Don't take bribes
9. Don't oppress strangers
10. Every seventh year, (the Schmidtah year) rest your fields and

labors and donate to the poor and to the wildlife.

11. Keep the seventh day holy, and rest and refresh

12. Don't even *speak* the name of other gods

13. Sacrifice the first of your first fruits to the temple and don't

participate in fertility-cult practices

14. God is sending an angel to keep you in the way, and bring

you into the place he has prepared

15. If you do all he says, God, will be an enemy to your enemies

and an adversary to your adversaries

16. God's angel will take you into the midst of your enemies and

will cut them off

17. Do not bow down to their gods, nor serve them, nor do after

their works: but you will utterly overthrow them and quite

break down their images

18. Serve God. Then, there will be no miscarriages, none baren in

    your land, and the number of your days will
be fulfilled

19.   God's fear will go before you and destroy all
those people you

    come to, so your enemies turn their backs to
you

20.   God will send hornets before you and drive
your enemies out

    before you; he will drive them out slowly over
a year's time,

    so the land won't be desolate and become
overrun by wild

    beasts until you are slowly increased and
inherit the land

21.   The land's inhabitants will be delivered into
your hands, and

    you shall drive them out before you; make no
covenant with

    them nor their gods (it will be a snare to you!)

The inhabitants in number 21—in this case, your parasitic enemies or demons—will lose strength and you will eventually cripple them physically, emotionally, and even spiritually because through your balance and good health you will have great power. Your intention to help or be nice to them may initially be one coming from a place of intended kindness, but the end result can still be terribly cruel and damaging to them and to yourself. Still, sometimes things we feel like should be done to be nice must happen for justice to be served. Not everything that seems nice is actually nice. Nice does not mean what you think it means. Am I saying never do anything kind for anyone? No. I'm saying don't take away opportunities for another's growth, and become discerning of those who truly need a little help from others and who needs to not be there at all. You need help too, you know, in some ways. Only you can help you first, and you should but then help from your own resources to help others, don't assume you can dip into someone else's basket to do more for someone else. That's not your job, nor is it right or good.

Building a healthy and balanced natural food diet is simple to do once you learn what to look for. I'll start at the very beginning, and we'll cover the most common aspects. As with everything in life, there will be the rare exception to the rule; but *don't* automatically jump to the conclusion that *you* are the exception.

I will reference everything as though I am talking to and giving advice to myself and referring to my own situation as always unless I specify otherwise. You are more than welcome to do the same and apply these things with any special modification you know you need. The point is to tailor the information to your situation. If you are unsure of any of these things, it's best to work with someone local, with proper training in this area. You don't want to mess this up!

One of the most important things to understand when discussing anything to do with food is self-control. Another word for self-control is temperance. For some, this may mean being able to know what foods to say "no" to, or knowing when your body has been satisfied, or knowing when to stop eating before the food does damage (Note: it's much earlier than you think), or knowing when you're restricting yourself too far and too much and causing a different kind of damage.

We don't have to look farther than to Paul for an example about temperance in the New Testament. First, let's first define *sedition*. Brittanica.com says that *sedition* is "a crime against the state" (see the webpage https://www.britannica.com/topic/sedition). This is usually done by organizing or encouraging opposition to government like in speech or writing. And *that* is what Paul was being accused of. [22]

There was a public speaker named Tertullus and he was jealous of Paul's popularity among the people. The high priest took Tertullus up to see the governor Felix and told him, basically, "Look, we've enjoyed a lot of peace and quiet under your reign, and now here comes Paul stirring up the Jewish people and he's trying to cause a riot against the government." They hold a trial, but all they can figure out is that there's some sort of disagreement regarding gospel doctrine and there was no sign of sedition.

Felix figured that if he let Paul go though, he's going to upset the Sanhedrin people in the land and there could be a riot or even a rebellion. He was also worried that Paul would get tired of house arrest and offer him a bribe, which Felix had been known in the past to take. Felix had even stolen his wife Drusilla, Herod Agrippa I's daughter, from another man when she was just sixteen. For the next two years, he kept calling Paul in, hoping for a money bribe. Instead, he always got an earful about his mortality and even a lesson on temperance (or self-control) and a coming judgment. This made Felix tremble in fear and alarm, and he repeatedly asked Paul to go away, and he'd call him back later.

Can we relate to Felix in regard to our own self-control—or in relation to food? Perhaps we push those feelings under the rug, or under a piece of cake, some ice cream, or a bag of chips. We'll deal with that later (or not at all), right? Meanwhile, our cells keep wasting away and dying, eventually shaving a potential ten, twenty, thirty years or more off a normal healthy, even robust life? Someone says the words *vegetable* or *salad,* and we want to say "You, go away now, I'll deal with you later!" But we must learn self-discipline, and not just with food. Still, it's a great place to start. And since we mentioned vegetables, that's a great place to start talking about one of my favorite subjects: foods!

If you're already familiar with my second book on hydration, *"Fountain of Living Water"*, you already know *that's* the most important place to start, even before food. Hopefully, you have already mastered that skill. In *this* book, we'll be covering fruits and vegetables, whole grains, proteins, healthy oils in moderation, drinking water and herbal teas, staying active, and quality of foods. As you know by now, though, being properly hydrated can completely change food needs and help the deep healing of poor health, so be sure to do that first!

Fruit is a food source that is probably one of the easiest and quickest broken down in the stomach and absorbed through the intestines, after water. Water and, in general, fruits will clear a well-functioning stomach after no more than twenty minutes. Please note that this can be complicated by illness, injury, or blockages. Of course, you should consult your healthcare providers about these things and seek treatment as needed.

Different fruits create different levels of energy as they're being broken down by our system. Some will burn shorter and others longer, like the difference between burning paper and hardwood. Some fruits will burn hotter in the body and others cooler. Also, some will leave behind an acidic ash and others an alkaline ash as it exits the body through the large intestine.

There is so much to know regarding this one simple aspect of how foods relate within and to the body. A whole book could cover this one topic alone. Plus, this does not apply to fruits only, but also to vegetables, grains, meat, oils, seeds, and more. All foods. All *life*.

How recently a food was harvested also influences how much life source is available for our body to break down and create usable energy; all foods have life sustaining resources for the body to break down. It is not the nutrients but the life force that gives us the life *resources*. This is often confused with the false concept of what we think the word *nutrient* means. Any reference to *nutrition* or *nutrient* should be understood as "life source" instead.

Nutrition refers to *how* the nutrients in food are *used*. Just because you eat a good diet doesn't mean you're always getting good nutrition. Each person's body chemistry is going to make all the difference in whether food is going to help your health or be detrimental.

Let's define what a fruit is and what it is not. Fruits are defined by the type of plant they come from as well as the part of the plant that they are. Merriam-Webster.com says *fruit* is:

1. (a) a product of plant growth (such as grain, vegetables, or cotton)

    (b) i. The usually edible reproductive body of a seed plant especially one having a sweet pulp associated with the seed

(b) ii. A succulent plant part used chiefly in a dessert of sweet course

(c) A dish, quantity, or diet of fruits

(d) A product of fertilization in a plant with its modified envelopes or appendages

2. offspring, progeny (fruit of the womb)
3. (a) The state of bearing fruit (A tree in fruit)

(b) The effect of consequence of an action or operation: product, result (the fruits of our labor, the fruits of victory)

4. OFFSPRING, PROGENY – fruit of the womb
5. The state of bearing fruit

   a. A tree in fruit
   b. The effect of consequence of an action or operation: PRODUCT, RESULT – the fruits of our labor, the fruits of victory

Collins.Dictionary.com defines *fruit* as "something which grows on a tree or a bush and which contains seeds or a stone covered by a substance that you can eat."

Britannica.com includes plants like vines, and even some grains and grasses. Biblically, fruit is a reference (in my favorite *Strong's Concordance*) to earnings, fruits, offspring, price, produce, product, results, and reward.

Back to the theme of self-control for a moment. An ancient list was given in two parts. The first part gave a list of virtues associated with living a life devoted to serving the self: a worldly "me first" kind of attitude that leads to self-destruction and that is natural for humans. The second part of the list shows us what grows naturally from those being led supernaturally by the Spirit of God and being marked by the "fruit of the Spirit." Two of those second list items are found in Galatians: gentleness and again, self-control. [23] These are among some of the most highly desired fruits of all! Just like breaking down and assimilating foods in the body, self-control brings us greater health, happiness, and power.

So now we know what *fruit* is and what it's not, let's start with how fruit relates to hydration, which was covered more thoroughly in *"Fountain of Living Water."* Not all fruits are the same. Some are more acid-forming and others more alkaline-forming. This does not mean the fruit is acidic or alkaline but has to do with how it breaks down in the body as it goes through the digestive process, is broken down, and what's left over. It's like the ash that's left over after intense heat consumes wood in a fire.

Remember, it is not the nutrients but the breaking down process that gives us energy needed for life in the body. Some fruits are sweeter, some more astringent, and they all break down at different levels of heat and energy that they produce. Some burn hotter and others cooler, just like wood. Some things burn up very quickly, some very slowly and thus produce different levels or heat or energy. Since we're talking first about fruits that are more hydrating and cooling to the body, let's list which are the *most* cooling from the most to least of the alkaline forming fruits.

ALKALINE FORMING HYDRATION FRUITS

- Blackberries
- Persimmons, Raspberries, Papaya, Pineapple
- Watermelon, Cantaloupe, Honeydew
- Blueberries, Apples, Cherries, Apricots
- Avocados, Olives (green), Banana, Pears, Peaches

This list is not all-inclusive. It covers the most basic, common hydrating fruits we use in the modern world from the grocery stores. But even though these are hydrating, they could make some people's health worse. For example, if the body's sugars are already high, some or all of these fruits might not be recommended to eat or should not be eaten after certain times of the day, or at all, depending on where all your body's levels are until they get evened back out.

In general, food can be easy, but it's specific to each individual, especially those with health issues. Having a trained specialist in nutrition to help you is highly recommended. You could throw off your body's chemistry and hormones very quickly and easily by eating the wrong things, or even the right things in the wrong order.

As tempted as we may be, we can't rely on the current medical industry for help starting out on the right foot for nutrition. A single four-hour class on nutrition is not enough training to put a scratch into all one must know just on fruits alone to understand the impacts on health and wellness. It's not their wheel house. That's not their fault. Just don't expect an apple to be a broccoli or vice versa.

Anyone who tells you food doesn't make a difference, or says that you can't change your acid-alkaline balance or your hormones have no idea what they don't know about what they don't know. Get out of there fast! (You can be really knowledgeable about some things and not at all about others.) There are places and people to whom you can go for help, and, in my experience, you're not going to find all your help in one place anyway. Don't let that intimidate you.

Contrary to popular belief, you can't just eat all the fruit you want, either. It will throw off your body's balance. Just like with farming, if you keep putting the same plant into your soil, eventually you *will* reach too much of a good thing, and it will ruin the soil, and nothing will grow well there until you rebalance the soil's pH and add variety again. Your crops won't be fruitful. It's the same with too much acidity or alkalinity in your body.

In the book of Peter there's another witness to the definition of fruits and self-control. When we lack self-control, we physically suffer. We are urged to stop over-indulging in the ways of eating and living that the world is teaching us, which ironically are destructive to health and true happiness. He even mentions how everyone will think you're weird if you're not joining in on the excess rioting with them, overindulging in luxuries, etc. [33]

Another story shares the importance of maintaining our body as a pure and clean receptacle. Scientists are now realizing that the body's DNA strands hold more than merely genetic coding. DNA is actually an antenna, like a radio antenna! It can send and receive messages between us and our Creator. A dirty or broken antenna is either not going to get a good signal or not get one at all. If we're not careful, it might even be tuned to a wrong channel.

God cannot dwell in an unholy temple (or, in other words, if your body is dirty inside and all clogged up), his signal cannot get through. No signal means no entry into his kingdom. How do we help keep our antenna clean? We're told we should be humble and it is easy to misjudge others as not being what we think being humble is but we must be very careful that we are not judging someone falsely as not being humble either. The best thing to do is to worry about our own selves and using God's standard for what humble is and isn't since it is his measuring tool in the first place anyway. Worrying about if someone else's level of humbleness may get us in trouble, especially if we don't truly understand the full measure of what it actually is. Since we don't know a person's heart or their intentions nor their perspectives, we can't really know for sure.

We are to be submissive and gentle, easy to entreat, full of patience, long-suffering, temperate in all things—ahh... *there's* that self-control again—and on and on; all the good stuff. [24] But we are made from dirt. Our physical form comes from the earth; and this is part of why we must learn to maintain our *inner* soil, become a master gardener, just as a diligent farmer would tend to his fields, if we are to have a good harvest.

You may have noticed that grapes and strawberries were not on the list above. While they contain a lot of water, they are also very astringent. If you tend to be a person with drier skin, for example, this can be very harmful and drying to the body because digesting strawberries and grapes will tend to break down the oils in your body. If dryness is already a struggle, this will only tend to make things worse. However, those who tend to have naturally oily or greasy skin, more astringent fruits may actually be very beneficial to you, depending on where your carbohydrate and other levels are in the body. If it's high enough, it may be best to avoid fruits until back in balance.

If you don't have the faith to incorporate new ideas and ways of doing things, you'll never know the feeling of acquiring that virtue. Virtue leads to knowledge, and knowledge to... wait for it... temperance or what? Which is also known as self-control... which is followed by patience, then brotherly kindness, eventually godliness, charity, humility, and finally, diligence. [35] You must practice a *lot* in order to be diligent at something.

The opposite of diligence is idleness, neglect, ignorance, and slothfulness. There was a boy, once sweet and good, who met with a tragedy in his life. Exposed to grown-up things far beyond his understanding and then left vulnerable to attack after attack, he very quickly slipped away into a very dark place. His psyche broken, his spirit shattered, fractured, and exposed, he began to fill with great darkness.

This darkness became compounded by poor food choices and eating habits, which further raised his anger, hatred, and acidity levels to alarming heights, and it seemed no one was able to help the lad. You see, he did not have the want or desire to free himself, believing the falsehoods he thought to be real: about food, his experiences, and himself. He even exposed himself to demonic influences, falsely believing that it gave him great power and authority over others. He was not able to see that stealing and taking from others (rather than having self-control) does not give you power, but truly makes you weak.

Bad foods do this to our system. We feel good for a moment but then need another *fix*. Much like any other drug, the brain becomes used to the repetition and begins to ignore the signals the body sends to the brain about what's happening to it, which is why drug addicts quickly move on to harder and harder drugs: to get the shocking rush in the brain again.

It was no different for this child, Gerald. He became extremely rebellious, filled with deep, depths of terrifying darkness, and began to prey on others, trapping them along with him in his own personal hell. He was not consciously aware of this initially and felt it was "who I am and how I have always been." Because this started so young and Gerald had stayed so focused on the darkness, he forgot being any other way.

He was molded and emotionally, mentally, and even spiritually tortured. The internal screams of his soul crucified the hearts of those around him who could hear, feel, and discern them but they knew not how to help him. Yet, even into his adulthood, he had no desire to even consider that he had the power to ask for help and begin taking actions to get himself free from the dark prison within his own mind.

The boy continued to eat food that weakened his body and cause him to think the things and still believe the thoughts and false beliefs he had grown up with. He allowed his captors and tormentors power over him rather than make the step towards his own liberation. But he is next to heal. His time has come. He can free himself. And so can you.

The mind is a powerful thing. It can repair itself; it can remold itself because it is so pliable. I, myself, had a large amount of brain damage after several traumas—even a stroke while being bedridden for a long period of time. Some things can be harmful, even if they seem at the time to be good things.

Let's look at some revelations that science has been starting to find really true. Take tobacco, for example. Mankind was told that tobacco is not for the body, not for the belly, and not for man at all. It's to be used as an herb for *bruises* only, and for sick cattle to ingest. The most important detail is to use it with *judgment* and *skill* for these purposes alone, so that means if you're going to use it at all, you'd better learn to do it the right way and from someone who knows how.

Don't smoke it, don't vape it, don't and chew it if you want to enjoy healthier days ahead. There may seem to be some benefits you think you might be enjoying from tobacco use; however; I think you will find there are better, healthier things that you can use that will bring even better outcomes for you without the health risks. This not only applies to yourself but affects those around you as well. This is where someone skilled in plants, foods, and holistic training can be of great aid in finding what works best for you.

There has been a lot misunderstood about the meaning of the word *wine*. A thousand years ago, alcohol content in beer was almost zero percent, but today you can find high levels of alcohol in everything from wine to beer to carbonated beverages and energy drinks, easily accessible to anyone.

In biblical times, *wine* usually referred to grape juice, which has been found to be very good for the heart. Psalms 104:15 notes that wine "maketh glad the heart of man, and oil to make his face shine, and bread which strengtheneth man's heart." Which is to say: the grain was processed in a healthy way and was very different from what can be bought in stores today. It would give you strength back then. Now, that's questionable. The oils were cold pressed and local. They were eaten quickly and not after they'd become rancid from a little heat exposure. And the wine was also processed and utilized more freshly or with lighter fermentation. There's a big difference, in other words, between the food of the gods and the foods of the world today. Which one are you going to put into your body?

I love the story of Daniel in the Bible. I think he was a man after the manner of my own heart. I am fascinated with the entire book of Daniel, and one day I would love to sit down in heaven with him and have lunch. What a conversation we might have! For those unfamiliar with the Daniel's story, let me briefly share:

In the third year of King Jehoiakim's reign in Judah, King Nebuchadnezzar came and laid siege on Judah, and God gave Jehoiakim and the land over to Nebuchadnezzar. The king asked his righthand man, Ashpenaz, to bring some of the children from Israel to the palace to teach them Nebuchadnezzar's ways. He wanted "children in whom was no blemish, but well favored, and skillful in all wisdom, and cunning in knowledge, and understanding science, and such as had ability in them to stand in the king's palace, and whom they might teach the learning and tongue of the Chaldeans. [38] Kind of like what the colonizers did to the Native American children when they came and took over America. Took their children, took their culture, and made them Chaldean—oops! I mean, English.

The king set aside some of his very own food and wine for these children to eat and to drink for three years so that at the end of this time, the children could stand before the king.

Four of these children were from Judah, including Daniel. Daniel spoke up and asked that he not be made to defile himself with the king's food because he knew it to be damaging to the body. [25] He asked Ashpenaz to do a test just for ten days and see if they looked better or healthier than the kids eating the king's food and wine.

Ashpenaz was worried that Daniel and the other children would actually look sicker and weaker after that time, and then he'd lose his head when the king got angry. So, Ashpenaz did the test secretly. The four children of Judah ate pulse (a combination of seeds and nuts) and water, while the rest of the children were fed the king's food and wine.

"And at the end of the ten days, their countenances appeared fairer and fatter in flesh than all the other children which did eat the portion of the king's meat." [26] So the servants of the king got rid of the king's portion of food and fed all the children the pulse and water. At the end of their education, none of the children were found wiser in understanding and in matters of wisdom than Daniel and the other children of Judah. These four kids were even "ten times better than all the magicians and astrologers in all [Nebuchadnezzar's] realm. [27] What you eat and drink—and where it comes from—does matter. Even who grew it matters; did you know?

Are your food growers local? Hopefully, you grow your own food. But if not, do the food growers in your area know and use the best growing practices? Not the ones of the world, the commercial practices, but the natural laws of nature and what's in the best, highest interest of nourishment for the body and the soil. Are packaging and handling practices contaminating or supporting your ultimate health, or are they putting profits and convenience first? Keep processing as minimal as possible and do "plant to plate" as much as you can.

One of the biggest, most important things you should know and understand is the true definition of moderation in *all* things. Some days moderate is going to look different than other days, depending on where the body chemistry is at that time. As you begin healing yourself deeply through food (so your physical form can support and maintain the changes), you can begin to heal the emotional scars. Not only will your body begin to change, but so will your mind. The right foods won't make the healing changes for you, you must still take additional action towards healing injuries and trauma, but foods will support you as you go through the process of healing.

When the Pharisees asked Jesus why he wouldn't receive them with their baptism, seeing that they were keeping the whole law as they saw it, he told them that they were not keeping the whole law. If they had been, *they* would have received *him*, because he is the one who gave them the law. He couldn't receive them because it didn't do them any good keeping the old law in partiality while believing it was full nor accepting him.

Then Christ told the Pharisees, "Neither do men put new wine into old bottles: else the bottles break, and the wine runneth out, and the bottles perish: but they put new wine into new bottles, and both are preserved." (Wine makers know that when you make wine you must put it into a new container because old ones are no longer strong enough to withstand the curing process and will burst under the pressure. This is why you put new wine into new bottles.)

So, what is this all about? Is it about the wine or the bottles? Actually, it's not about either! During Jesus's life, there were people of the law who did a lot of good things outwardly for all to see, but many of them had very hard hearts and were prideful. They were constantly attacking Jesus and looking for any little thing they could find to tear him down. They didn't like how popular Jesus was becoming. In their eyes, Jesus's actions threatened and broke the laws of the land, but Christ lived a perfect life and actually came to fulfill the law, which he did.

People asked Jesus why the Pharisees fasted but the disciples didn't, and he instead asked them how the children of the bridechamber could fast, while the bridegroom was with them? He told them that they could not, as long as they had the bridegroom with them but the time will come when the bridegroom will be taken from them, and on that day, they will fast.

If fasting puts us in the right mindset and in alignment with God's will for our greatest joy and happiness *and* it demonstrates our sacrifice, what related to food are we working on to get us there? What can we put on the altar? A sacrifice of something we *think* we love for something that gives us back so much more in return. What are we willing to give up for good health? Sometimes, when we give up that something we loved as a sacrifice—maybe a habit of eating after 7:00 p.m., eating processed foods, or not eating regularly scheduled meals at the same time every day—it can leave a hole in us, a tear.

We might be tempted to patch the (metaphorical) hole in our own body as an easy, quick repair. But no one sews a patch of unshrunken cloth on an old garment. If you do, the new, stronger piece will pull away from the old and make the tear worse.

In the Bible, Christ did not come to patch Judaism up with a new piece of material but to fulfill it; to *fulfill* Judaism. His role is not to plug the holes but to redeem. *Redeem.* His role is to bring back what once was, before the harm; *before.* The Pharisees were living their lives and the ideas that they were trying to teach by putting new wine into old bottles, causing their bottles to burst and waste the spilt wine.

When we change our eating habits and eat the right way, as he taught us, we become like a new wine! But he does not—and cannot—put us back into our old vessel. We must be freed from the prison of the old residue that lingers on in our old vessel. We must have something new contain us; something stronger that can hold, protect, and contain our newfound strength, vigor, and vitality. Healing deeply can be much like this.

If we strive to be like Christ and are to become like him, should we not then strive for ultimate purity, cleanliness health-wise, and in holiness? For example, it is comparable to being worthy to be a bishop. What should a bishop be? And then, how can we apply that to foods?

First, a bishop must be blameless, the husband to only one wife, and vigilant. That's dedication right there. Have you looked up that definition of *vigilant* lately? Wow. He must also be sober—there's that self-control again!—of good behavior (naturally), apt to teach, not given to wine or drunkenness, and not a violent bully. A bishop should also not be greedy of filthy lucre but be patient, not a brawler, and not covetous. [39]

I recently attended a mental health fair where there was in attendance quite a few ladies whose faces were all bruised up, who had "fallen," – which I knew was code for "in an abusive relationship"— and they knew I knew. And these ladies were resigned to their respective situations because they each believed there was no way out. I wanted to grab them all up and take them away with me and nurture them and teach them a better way. But all I could do is give them some information with the hope that they would follow up on it (or that their friend who brought them would). Which is to say: I cannot express how essential self-control is in basically *everything*!

Likewise, don't wish that you had what someone else has, does, or is. Just be authentically *you*. You are amazing enough just as you are. Nothing is as magical or unique as you; do not try to be someone else or something you never truly were in the first place. People can read that right off the bat and what they want is truly, the authentic you!

One of my heroes is King Solomon, the wise, ruler, and judge. I admire how much he loved God and wanted to do right by him. In those days, there was not a temple built, there was no altar for sacrifices, there was no wall around the city. The people had to go up into the high places of the land to offer up their sacrifices.

While Solomon was in Gibeon to make a sacrifice to God there (it was considered the great high place), he was said to have offered up a thousand burnt offerings. Was this literal or figurative and was this all at once or over time? I don't know for sure, but either way: it would be a lot. Then, God came to Solomon in a dream by night. God told Solomon to ask him what he was going to give to the man. Not knowing what to do in his new role as king (because he was replacing King David) and being so young, Solomon asked God instead to give him an understanding heart so he could discern between good and bad. Who could judge such a great people as God's chosen?

Solomon's request pleased God so much that he also gave Solomon his other gift anyway. After all, the young man had not asked God for a long life for himself, nor riches, nor for his enemies' lives, but for discernment and fair judgment. Can you imagine tickling God's heart so delightfully? I love thinking about that a moment. I bet that's one of God's favorite memories!

Like Solomon, when we do not know where to turn or how to move forward, we can also receive inspiration in relation to foods and any other areas of our lives where we might need additional guidance. We may have researched as much as we can, and studied which providers are available in our area, ways to grow our own foods with our unique situations and come to a point where we need a little more insight than we have access to or just to confirm that we have made the right choice to proceed with. Keeping our antennae clean and receptive we can receive answers to these questions. We can make our own sacrifices to show our dedication and commitment to act on the answers or knowledge we may receive. It may not be a thousand burnt offerings on the top of a mountain but you can think of something that would be a pleasing demonstration of giving up something precious to you that would be pleasing to God.

At some time during Solomon's rein, two women who each recently gave birth three days apart from each other and happened to be living in the same house. One night, one mother accidentally laid on her baby, and it died during the night. She got up at midnight, soon realizing what had happened and switched her dead baby for the other woman's living baby. The next morning, the second woman figured out that the babies had been switched and she had the first woman's dead baby. Because they couldn't settle their conundrum themselves, they ended up before King Solomon.

Both women claimed the baby was hers. The king asked for a sword and said to divide the living child in two and give half to each woman. Because she loved her son so much, the real mother begged him to give the whole baby to the other woman and not to kill him. The mother of the dead baby said "Let it be neither mine nor yours but divide it."

Using his good judgment, King Solomon awarded the living baby back to its real mother, who wanted to spare its life. The news spread through all of Israel, of course. Everyone had so much respect for the king, for they saw he had much wisdom. [40]

What a sensational story! It demonstrates how Solomon's gift was used in such a complicated way that a young boy would not have had the wisdom to determine on his own knowledge or experience and gives us hope that we too can receive answers to the things that plague us in our lives. Sometimes I think we feel like the woman who lost their baby in the middle of the night because of something that was our own fault in relation to foods, our mismanagement of them, and the health issues we end up struggling with because we did not use wisdom sooner. It can feel difficult giving up foods that we've overused, abused, and maybe even worshipped.

Other times, I think we feel like the mother of the living child who was robbed and discovered her babe missing and in the hands of a grieving person. In the arms of someone who will stop at nothing to live in her fairytale world pretending her child is still living. We scramble desperately to get back what was once ours, hoping professionals can help us get it returned to us whole, and unharmed. Or maybe we are even the people nearby, watching the story unfold of either of these two women, or someone who is struggling to learn how to use food more wisely, wondering at the possible outcomes or who is lying.

Could we be King Solomon, sitting on his judgement seat, looking over the information, pondering, weighing the details, praying to judge rightly, receiving confirmation and taking action. Only you will know which you are at each pivotal moment of your food healing journey.

Gerald could have used a King Solomon.

His parents could have used having King Solomon's wisdom in how to help Gerald, in how to use proper nutrition to help begin to balance him out more while they tried to find him more and better help. The right kind of help. His parents probably also could have used better nutritional support for themselves as well with all the stress they were under during Gerald's entire life growing up. You can't go back and change the past *but* you *can* learn from it. It doesn't even have to be your own past. You can usually see a part of your story in every single person that you meet. A solution or even a cautionary tale.

Remember Gerald. Learn from his past. Create a better food future. Create if for yourself, for your family, for your community.

Chapter 4
Antiuchus

A WOMAN NAMED ANTIUCHUS found herself in several situations that brought about great compassion and feeling in me due to her life trials, misconceptions, and health precepts. She believed very strongly that she was right in her thinking and was quick to discern and judge a situation in milliseconds. With the tenacity of a bulldog in a fight (and even to the point of her own detriment), she would hold on to her own ideas, already sure that she knew how to eat healthy.

She and her family ate rice, beans, veggies, and salads. Seemingly, there's nothing wrong with these ingredients. She was completely closed off to even considering, let alone actually creating, more balance in her family's diet. She sought ways to help maximize their budget while simultaneously trying to minimize emotionally traumatic situations going on in her family. She *said* that she was looking for new solutions but was unwilling to hear or even experiment upon any of them offered to her.

Antiuchus prepared her family's meals with these foods, but there were mostly grain carbs from the rice with a few tiny flecks of finely diced sweet peppers (a nightshade plant) in small enough quantity to be considered a *hint* of light seasoning. She used in her dishes an inflammatory amount of cheese and nothing that would truly sustain life and good health for very long.

I could see where some easy changes could be made that would not have cost her family any more money: there were no complete proteins included, and this type of diet lent itself to eating lots of processed sugar at their meals, blissfully in denial of the harm they were inflicting upon themselves and still wondering why the children were always so hungry.

Antiuchus and her family choose to keep things as they were, and I stood back and watched everything in their lives slowly disintegrate around them, including their mental health. It was really difficult to watch, but I had offered an easy, affordable solution that could be easily implemented. They made their choice, and my hands were tied from rendering any further assistance.

You can choose to stay where you are, or you can take a chance and *MOVE*!!! Antiuchus did not see or realize the danger her health was in, or that of her family's though she did see they were in trouble. Even after being warned by someone with an outside vantage point, able to see what she could not—or *would* not—she chose to remain blind (and *right,* if only in her mind - *hello cognitive dissonance* - again).

At some point, we all have to ask ourselves, "Do I want to be right, or do I want to get better?" You decide, and even if you decide that you want to get better, it does not mean you were wrong in the first place. You see, when you make a decision to *do* something, even if it's different from what you were doing before, you are right about deciding to even try it. You choose it, so it's still right, even if all you get is a learning experience out of it.

Be adventurous; try new things! And give yourself some grace. Don't expect lettuce to be ice cream. They're not the same. They're very different in flavor, texture, color, scent, vibration, life force—everything! If you expect lettuce to be ice cream or ice cream to be lettuce, you'll be disappointed every time, my friend. Every time.

Give things a chance to just be what they are, be just what they were created for, and don't focus on what they're not or you'll wish they were instead. You'll miss the full measure of amazingness of an experience because you're not present, you're focusing your attention and heart elsewhere, on other things. Do not covet, and you'll end up with something *way* better for *you*. Stay focused on your goal.

After Christ's resurrection, the number of disciples eventually multiplied. The Grecians started complaining against the Hebrews because the Grecians felt that their widows were being neglected in daily welfare acts. So, the original twelve disciples called for the Grecians to look amongst themselves and find seven men known for their honesty who were filled with the Holy Ghost and wisdom so that these local men could be called to these ministering positions and there would be enough people to help.

The Grecians chose a man named Stephen, who was full of faith and the Holy Ghost, along with six others. These men were called to their work, set apart, and then began their tasks. Stephen was full of faith, he acted, he had power, and he did great wonders and miracles among the people. He was so filled with light and power that when several groups of people brought up disagreements with him, they "were not able to resist the wisdom and the spirit by which he spake." These disciples were living the true laws of health and were given light and increased wisdom that has been promised to those who keep these laws. [29]

You're probably wondering why I've mentioned Stephen here; probably to reference helping the poor and needy, you're thinking, but no. I'm more thinking about his character and good qualities and relating that to our foods—what we are putting into our bodies—and how that relates to the poor and needy *cells* in our bodies that need nourishing. Let's extrapolate on that a bit.

Stephen's calling came about by the notice of the people in the community that included members who were struggling. These widows (the Grecians who were being neglected) were not getting what they needed, including services they could not do for themselves. So, the community was asked to find a person who was:

A. Honest

B. Close to the spirit of God

C. Wise

D. Someone who would take action

E. Filled with the power of faith

These are all powerful traits. What can we take away and apply to our nutrition with values like that? What would our stores, our food supply chains look like if they were run by those who were honest, faithful, wise, and took actions to have consumers' best interests at heart? What could we change personally to encourage that in our own lives, in our own diets, and in our food habits?

How much more energy we could have by being an 100% honest consumer or home grower of our own vegetables or fruits! What would happen if we began growing foods best for us by the Spirt and in adherence to nature's laws of healthy eating? How can we be wise in what and how we grow foods naturally in a way that sustains us and our family? Imagine the possibilities if we all worked together toward a common healthy food goal. Our bodies would strengthen and would grow to a point that an old, holey, broken vessel could no longer contain a being so filled with light and wholeness!

We would each require a new, whole, completely brand-new vessel. And *that* is what the old wine in new bottles is about: we must put new wine into new vessels.

Health issues aside, and still speaking generally while knowing there are always exceptions to any rule, fruits should generally be enjoyed earlier in the day. Only one or two servings are usually plenty, and combining multiple fruits together with increased frequency is going to provide better results than eating just one fruit by itself and another one later.

When in doubt, remember the Rule of 5. That's the minimum number you want to shoot for when mixing types of fruits or vegetables together. The more of one thing you combine, the more types of co-factors—a necessary ingredient that helps enzymes break down foods you eat—the body has available to help break down what you eat. So, the more types you consume, the more you'll get out of the food you eat. You'll feel more satisfied and fuller too!

Example 1: You could eat a salad made only of iceberg lettuce or only romaine, and all you're going to get is just that one little bit of nutrition.

Example 2: You make a salad with five or more types of lettuce in it, following the Rule of 5: maybe you use iceberg, romaine, green leaf, red leaf, arugula, or butter leaf, or even dandelion greens, parsley, and cilantro. Now, not only do your salad greens make a lot more salad—and last longer—you're going to be getting five or more different types of overlapping co-factors and thus the ability to break down and ingest a *LOT* more energy and good health out of that dish! As they say in Proverbs, "It shall be health to thy navel [belly], and marrow to thy bones." [30]

I'm getting ahead of myself again; we're talking about fruits. So, maybe you make a fruit salad to eat before you start on breakfast and from the list we grab and slice up some bananas, blueberries, raspberries, strawberries, and grapes; then squeeze some fresh lemon over it to liven it up a little bit. Wow! Now, it's more delicious; berries love berries! And following the Rule of 5, this fruit salad now has more antioxidants for the body and has multiple colors: red, white, and blue (or red, yellow, and blue) —the primary colors of the rainbow. Plus, all the various co-factors work together to give you a *lot* more bang for your buck.

Maybe you want to keep your fruit salad more tropical. You could use papaya, pineapple, mango, persimmon, and bananas with a squeeze of fresh lemon to liven it up. (A healthy liver likes a little fresh lemon on food from time to time. How much will depend on your digestive constitution and what your body needs and can handle. Too much lemon can make your heart palpitate, so use it wisely.)

From everything I have studied, been trained in, and experienced, you'll do well to stick to just one or two servings of fruit a day and get more of your plant needs from vegetables and greens. *In general,* you will get the best results this way, as long as you're basically healthy. If you have health issues, I recommend working with a professional trained in holistic nutrition to teach you the basics and get you closer to balanced again. It will be money well spent.

Remember, there's always the exception to the rule. And, if you're *really* sick, make sure you are working together with *all* your healthcare providers and keeping them all in the loop of what you're doing: medical, holistic, nutritional, etc. Everything is going to depend on *your* body's overall constitution, but don't make the mistake of using poor health as an excuse to get away with doing whatever you want to do instead of what's right for you.

Keep in mind: other influences and factors may also come into play and try to coerce or convince you to do things that are unhealthy for you. These may include parasites, bad bacteria, emotional trauma, bad habits, internal or outside influencers, susceptibility to persuasion from those who would lead you astray, and more.

NOTE: try to avoid eating the exact same food combinations every day. Variety in your diet will produce stronger and longer-term effects and eventually fill a larger wellness warehouse.

This may go without saying, but in an effort to be thorough and in case you need this information: once you have grown, locally harvested, picked, or purchased your fruit, wash it very thoroughly. These foods are grown outside in nature. There are birds and bugs climbing on it, particles from air pollution falling, and other dirty things happening to your produce. You don't know what is on that food.

If your food is picked by other workers who are out sweating in the heat, *that's* getting on the fruit and so are their allergies, coughing and sneezing fluids. And there is a lot of coughing and sneezing when you're out picking that all day. I've worked in the fields and orchards for a summer or two, and I've seen and experienced first-hand what goes on. It can't be helped. All that dust and dirt gets up your nose and between that and the heat you have to sneeze and cough a *lot*. It gets gross out there. *Please*, wash your fruits and vegetables really well before eating them even if you think the store misting them to keep them from wilting is enough. It's not.

The store-bought fruits that look all clean, shiny and polished? That's fake. Those fruits have been coated with either a wax (which may also be dyed) or will have some type of chemical or oil film that you shouldn't eat. It's there to make unripe fruit look ripe and *pretty*. You've got to get that washed off first, and that's not easy to do. Better to buy local or grow your own!

Maybe you're thinking "I'll just peel it, then." If you do that, you'll miss out on the super important enzymes in the skin, and enzymes are great in the war against cancer and other things. Buy local and tell your produce department you want 100% organic, non-waxed, non-coated produce. Your voice has power, and I invite you to speak up. If not for yourself, to help others who need this available to survive and those not able to speak up for themselves due to illness or immobility.

Large corporations know that each person who speaks up counts for 7,000 other people who feel the same way but did not speak up. It's true. Be the change. Ask for and buy and grow local foods. Your voice *matters*. And don't avoid doing it because you think someone else will, because they won't and they aren't. This depends on *you* and your voice. It's up to you. Act.

An important housekeeping matter: *always* wash your hands with *soap _and_ water* before preparing food or after using the bathroom or attending to other body grooming habits. You must use *both* soap and water. *EVERY* time. Regrettably, some people have not realized how much *not* doing this can contribute to the spread of bad bacteria and disease. It's a simple step to complete and doesn't cost much to do, especially compared to the cost of the illnesses created by not doing it.

Make sure you keep your kitchen and tools clean too, washing them after each use. Remember to rinse off all the soap residue. If there are still streaks or film, rinse a bit longer with plenty of clean, fresh water. When creating a fruit dish, try to make up just only what you will eat during *that* meal. It may take practice, but you'll get there. Once you cut or crush fruit, it starts breaking down and disintegrating much more quickly. Its nutritional and energy value disappears soon after.

Now on to vegetables and greens!

A lot of these same principles apply to vegetables as they do to fruits, so I'll just give you the short version here. The Rule of 5 means five or more types of veggies combined for higher absorption. Wash them really well; eat soon after harvest; eat 100% organic, non-GMO, non-coated foods; and keep your hands and work surfaces clean. Also, grow as much of your own food as possible.

On to which foods are the most beneficial, as promised in my previous book *"Fountain of Living Water,"*
198

and how food increases hydration absorption. For people with the weakest digestive systems, having your foods cooked—even salad—is ideal if you can. (If you think they have an iron stomach or a stomach of steel, let me tell you: it's not actually that strong. It's so sensitive that it shuts everything down and quits working at the slightest sign of trouble.)

This does not mean that people with the strongest digestive type should only eat raw foods all the time. Raw and cooked foods are both beneficial for different things. You need both. A good way to think of it is: raw foods clean and pull out of the body, and cooked foods feed and nourish the body. If you only eat raw foods, and you are only cleaning out the body and never nourishing it. In time, you will create weakness and depletion. In a manner of speaking, the body will become brittle.

Likewise, if you only nourish and never "clean out" the body's "house," things will eventually get clogged and backed up! Since neither scenario is desirable, both types of food are necessary. Your health level will determine how much of each your body needs and can and will tolerate. An expert can be beneficial in helping you figure this out if you have health challenges. You may not realize that some of your challenges might be health-related, so it might be a good idea to see a professional anyway and make sure. You don't know what you don't know—until you know. And then you know!

<u>COOKED VEGETABLES THAT HYDRATE:</u>

- Broccoli
- Lima beans
- Asparagus
- Brussels sprouts
- Green beans
- Onions
- Garlic
- Leeks
- Scallions
- Sweet potatoes
- Artichokes
- Baby corn
- Okra
- Eggplant
- Celery
- Zucchini

This is not an exhaustive list, but it covers the basics to help you get started.

I know you're wondering about other vegetables you don't see on the list, thinking to yourself, "But I love potatoes, carrots, or peas. They have healthy things about them. What about spinach and salads? So, first things first. The previous list focuses on hydration-increasing veggies. There is a *lot* more to basic nutrition, and its *way* more information than we can cover in one small book. That's why this is an area where working with someone trained in nutrition from a natural healing background is so important. Again, I highly encourage it.

Even if you feel pretty confident in your knowledge, like Antiuchus was, you don't know what you don't know. You may be surprised in what you learn, but wouldn't you rather know? If you go to someone and *don't* learn something new, chances are that you went to a person more medically trained, not someone trained in holistic nutrition, or you need someone with more advanced training than you have.

Similarly, beware of coaching others based on what you learned for (or about) yourself. Everyone has uniquely different body chemistry from what you have. What may be good for you may be dangerously unbalancing for someone else, and just because you can't see it on the outside or see an immediate result doesn't mean harm is not being done. Yes, even if you're blood-related and grew up in the same house, eating the same foods; even if you're identical twins.

<u>COOKED VEGETABLES THAT HYDRATE:</u>

<table>
<tr><td>

- Broccoli
- Lima beans
- Asparagus
- Brussels sprouts
- Green beans
- Onions
- Garlic
- Leeks

</td><td>

- Scallions
- Sweet potatoes
- Artichokes
- Baby corn
- Okra
- Eggplant
- Celery
- Zucchini

</td></tr>
</table>

What you don't know that you don't know about food interrelations and cross-reactions is the most problematic. The information I'm sharing in this book is very general in nature and is for relatively healthy people. Those with health conditions or illness should definitely coordinate their food plan (created by a nutritionist, a naturopath, or functional medicine provider) and their medical care plan so things can be put together in a way that works—with all the plans with food being a *high* priority.

Now, let's talk about those leafy greens. Leafy greens are another seemingly hydrating food. You are going to want to use your greens *cooked*. Some good greens include:

HYDRATING LEAFY GREENS

- Kale
- Spinach
- Swiss chard
- Bok choy
- Beet tops

- Collard greens
- Mustard greens
- Turnip tops
- Carrot tops

The majority of the time, these should be cooked. (*Most* people don't know this, so don't feel too badly if you didn't know either.) I'm not talking boiled to death. Let's be realistic: many of these leaves are quite delicate, aside from maybe the collard and mustard greens. A light blanching or steaming may be enough to deactivate the oxalates in them that block the body's ability to uptake and use calcium in the food. That's right. Go back and reread that: raw leafy greens can *block* calcium absorption.

Let me repeat: eaten raw, these leafy greens, block calcium. How important is that? Well, *VERY important*! Boil these plants, just like Brussels sprouts, to draw out the oxalates into the water, and then dump out the water. (You can save it if you like. Cool it off first and use is to water your plants or something, but don't drink it!) Cooked leafy greens can help you absorb your calcium from those foods, and the calcium, in turn, helps your cells use hydration better.

"But I put raw spinach (or kale or whatever) in my smoothies and I love it! It makes me feel better!" I can't tell you how many times I've heard this very statement. Of course you feel better—because you need more plants in your diet. I'm not taking your kale away. We're just going to change it a little tiny, tiny bit.

Cook the spinach, kale, or whatever. Then drain it, cool it, and pack it into an ice cube tray. Now, freeze it. Store the ice cubes in a freezer-safe container. Then, when you're ready to make your smoothie, add some of the green kale ice cubes to your blender in place of regular water ice cubes. They will be frozen, so your smoothie will keep cold, you will experience better absorption, and you won't even notice a difference in the taste. Make your smoothies, then return and report!

Spinach is fine-leafed, so it only needs to be barely blanched. It should still be bright green after cooking; if it's more olive, grey, or black, it's been overcooked. All the vitamins will have leaked out into the water, it won't taste very good, and the life force and nutrients will be missing.

Consider salad greens as another leafy green. Think of the leaf lettuces like butter leaf, romaine, bronze or red leaf. Even iceberg lettuce has a purpose: it has nutrients and is very hydrating. Other salad greens include green leaf, dandelion greens, watercress, arugula, herbs like parsley, cilantro, etc. As far as this goes, the same rules apply. Use the Rule of 5+ to increase absorption, cook (even lettuces!) to get more nourishment, eat raw to cleanse the body.

<u>HYDRATING LEAFY GREENS</u>

- Kale
- Spinach
- Swiss chard
- Bok choy
- Beet tops
- Collard greens
- Mustard greens
- Turnip tops
- Carrot tops

Here's a little-known fact about lettuce that you're going to love: if you have bad smelling body odor, *no* cream is going to *fix* or remedy that if the problem is coming from inside of you due to poor diet or too many antibodies. That's an internal problem, but it's easily fixed. Lettuce is like an "internal deodorant." If you smell yeasty, skunky, or like taco seasoning, that's *not* a natural body scent that indicates a mature body. That's the body's way of alerting you to an imbalance that needs correcting before it becomes even more dangerous. More lettuces, more cooked greens and hydrating vegetables may be in order! Remember nutritionists recommend to increase water intake too. Even consuming spices can require more hydration. Think of it like an internal sauna or spa—ohhh, so nice.

Consume these foods regularly and daily for maintenance, maybe even more than once a day in some cases until it gets under control. Then continue with maintenance. Remember: raw to cleanse, cooked to nourish. Raw should equal one serving for every two cooked servings each meal. Consider, too, are you eating greens with your breakfast?

OLIVE LEAVES

Here is just a nibble of an "'olive leaf'...plucked from the Tree of Paradise, a message of peace to us all." The message is: "Cease to be idle; cease to be unclean; cease to find fault with another; cease to sleep longer than is needful; retire to thy bed early, that ye be not weary; arise early, that your bodies and your minds may be invigorated. [43]

Healthy foods help hydrate and clean, and when we feel better, we can move better. When our insides are clean, we can think better and make better choices that ultimately not only will help us maintain good health but will also help us attain more bliss in life. If we want to feel good, be happy, and especially want to be able to enjoy this life we have to live a moderately balanced clean life as much as we possibly can. Each one of the twelve resources mentioned in the book "*Member Heal Thyself*" takes us one step—one layer—closer to that happiness we're looking for. Happiness is a conscious choice; it's a conscious effort. Like riding a bike: if you want to reach your destination, you'll have to start pedaling.

[1]

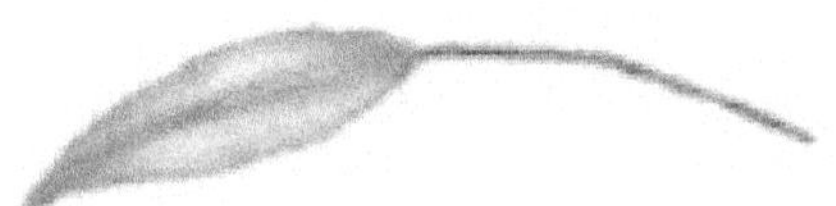

Ceasing to be idle is our first olive leaf and can be thought of as sitting on that bike pointed towards wellness but not pedaling, or not putting forth the effort. What matters is what you are making of *your* level of effort. It's not the *world's* standard of effort, nor is it possible to compare that to another person's level of effort or endurance during the effort. It cannot be measured against someone else's cup. We all have different measuring tools and mountains to overcome.

Stay consistent. Keep coming back to it, even if you feel you are starting over *again* for the millionth time! Because, whether you have realized it or not, each time you started, you've moved the starting line a bit closer to the goal. Each time you start *again* you are a little bit stronger. Each time you begin, you prove to yourself that you haven't given up on that goal, that dream. There's *power* in work.

[2]

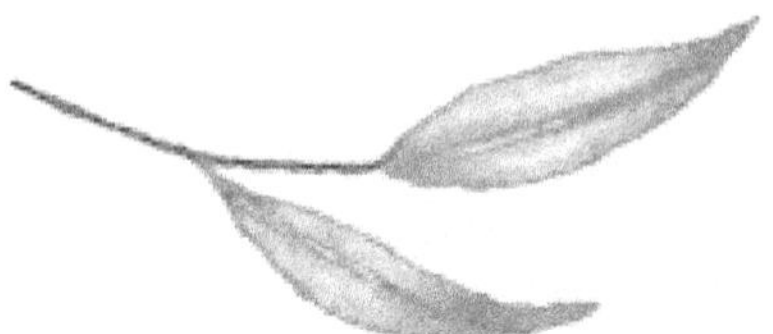

Being clean is vital to all areas of life: physical, mental, emotional, and spiritual. My second book, goes into the topic of water quite in depth, if you'd like a refresher: *"Fountain of Living Water."* It also includes some activities and recipes I think you'll really enjoy trying out. Being clean is also important to washing your foods before preparing and eating them.

How we grow our foods can be done in a "clean" manner as well and brings us far greater benefits. Yes, dirt is, well, *dirt-y* but there is a difference between soil that is whole and balanced and soil filled with bad bacteria and harmful organisms. Make sure your growing beds in your gardens have a healthy balance of good organisms in them to keep things in check. The same goes for our gut. A clean gut yields better brain balance and more clarity of thought, calmer emotions, and greater strength.

[3]

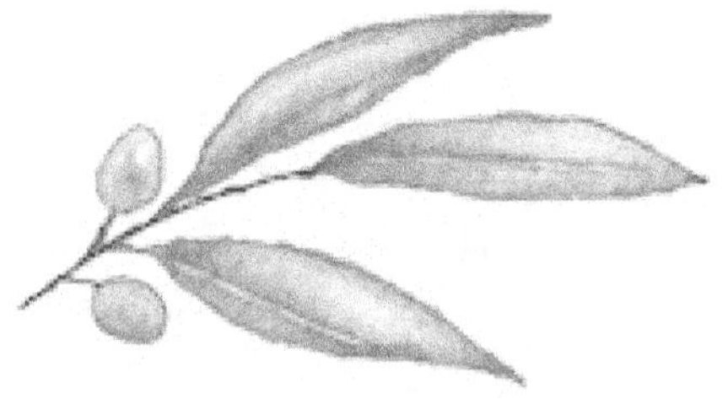

Finding fault with one another can fall into so many categories. Criticizing someone or something excessively drags us down to a lower vibration. Light has a very high vibration, as science has proven to us over and over. When we participate in criticizing others, we get dragged down lower and darker; we *become* lower and darker.

Way too often, especially on social media, we see so many are jumping in on the blame train, condemning this person or that for not liking one thing or another. We see bullying and physical, emotional, and spiritual attacks. How can we combat this? Opt out. Choose not to engage with it. Walk away. Fill your surroundings with the *opposite*. Be the light. Find things to give praise for, honest, specific and *sincere* praise.

Do this at least twice a day and see what starts to happen around you. Look for things, or create things, you can approve of. Chances are many others are hoping you will. Who or what can you recommend to others? Once you start to look and begin to do, you will begin to see or feel a shift in your environment.

[4]

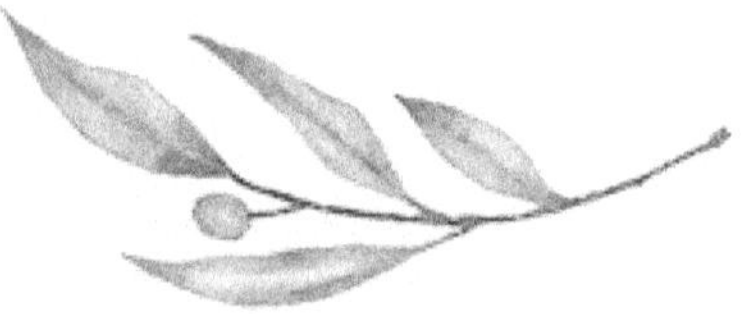

The next olive leaf is to stop sleeping longer than you need to. This topic is *so* important that I'll be covering this in depth in a future resource book. For now, in relation to

210

foods, know this: your body cannot produce a healthy microbiome in your belly if you don't eat the right amount and, the right quantities of foods that feed your gut flora. Your brain health is also linked to proper dietary nourishment and is tied to your gut. When one or the other is off—the gut, the brain, the diet, or sleep—one, two, three, or all four are affected.

Getting the right amount of sleep *and* at the right times of night has an effect on the quality of not only your sleep but also the proper sense of rest you crave. It can affect your emotions, behavior, and even how you're able to physically perform—whether it's working out, working at the office, or tending to your family or friends.

Sleeping too long may be a sign the gut is crying out for help. Many accidents, injuries, and mistakes can be chalked up to poor sleep habits and patterns. There are a lot of factors that are involved, but if you get to sleep by 9 p.m. every night and awaken between 6 a.m. and 8 a.m. the next morning (depending on what point you are at with your healing ritual point), you'll notice a really big difference not only in how you feel but in how you sleep *and* how you eat. That's right; I'll say it again. It *can* make a big difference in how you eat!

[5]

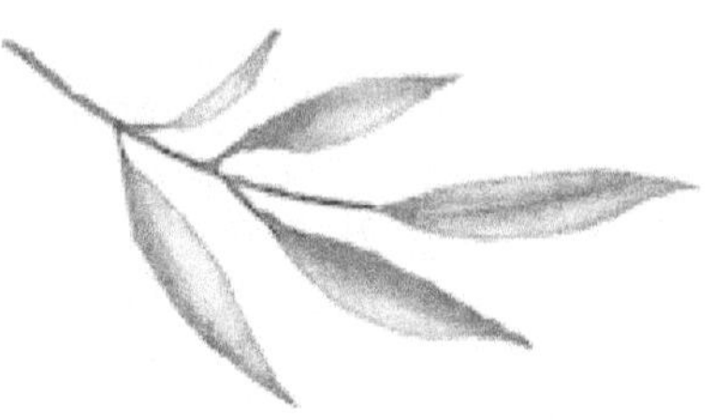

An olive leaf benefit comes from going to bed *early*: a secret to living healthier. Living healthier helps us feel happier and calmer and be more relaxed. We can enjoy the benefits of more hours of intense rest before midnight, and we can enjoy more happiness in all areas of our life. We make wiser choices, we handle our finances a little bit better, we eat things that honor our Creator and the wondrous forms he created for us to inhabit during this earth life experience.

I'll share more of some of the experiences I've had with this kind of sleep in a future resource book, but for now, the magic number for going early to bed is 9:00 p.m. Be competitive at rest; as one of my clients who struggles with rest says, "Be the best!" She says that shifts her perspective about it which really helps her make it a very important part of her day and week.

[6]

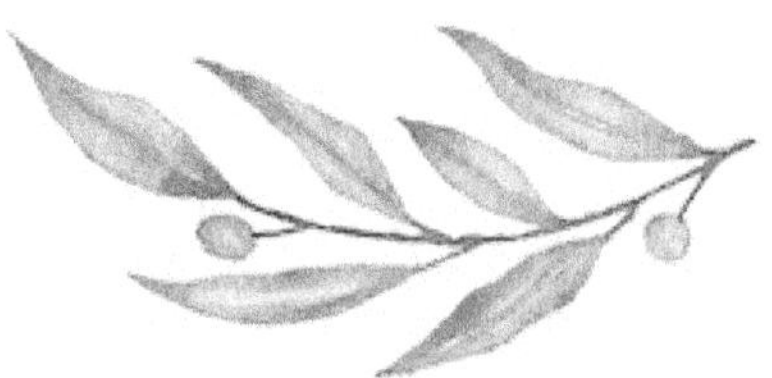

Waking up and getting out of bed *early* brings another olive leaf with a plethora of benefits to body, mind, and spirit. Not only does rising early help us avoid sleeping longer than is needful, it also helps us in regulating organs, glands, and even the entire nervous system. We can find mornings difficult for us when there is imbalance in the body, something we'll cover in a future resource book. When mornings are a struggle, we can use this as a sign there is more work to do with healing the gut, the microbiome, the brain, our foods, and our sleep patterns.

Even exercise, covered extensively in the next book, can affect our sleep, sleep patterns, and dietary choices—and vice versa. Exercise is a key link to all our health habits and patterns, and right now that may seem like a dream we cannot yet imagine.

[7]

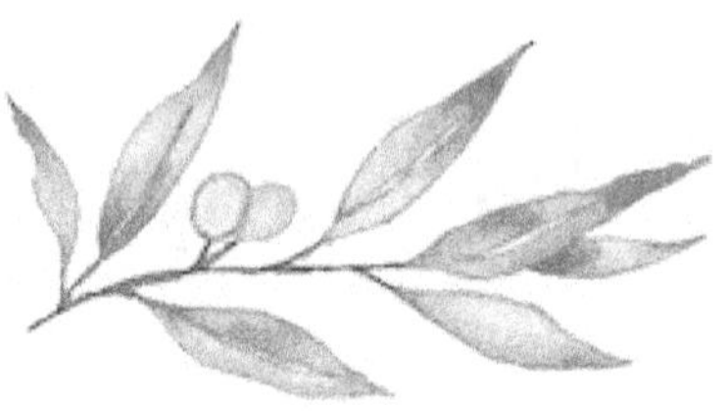

The final olive leaf is that if we do all of these things, we can look forward to our bodies and minds being invigorated; we can *expect* it. Remember vigor? It's physical or mental strength, energy or force, life force, life power, life strength. Vigor is the capacity for natural growth and, indeed, survival. It means feeling strong, whatever that means for you, and having enthusiasm for and, intensity for living.

Imagine that feeling of wanting to give up being so far gone from your mind and body that you can't even remember it anymore. *That's* what vigor should feel like: happiness, pure. This is not something that we will necessarily feel all the time, twenty-four hours a day, seven days a week. Like all of life's cycles, it will also ebb and flow. We will experience opposition in all things and even in this.

It's simple: you, but *better*. What could you do with a life full of vigor, a sense of meaningful purpose, and a full complete sense of happiness? When our insides are clean, we can think better and make better choices that ultimately help us maintain good health but *also* help us attain more bliss in life.

Chapter 5
Health

IN OLD ENGLISH THERE IS A word that is said to denote a healing power. This same word is proclaimed to offer a person deliverance. It is also known to bring a person, yes, even salvation. How can one single work be so powerful? It comes in a tiny little underdressed package that overdelivers and has more bang for its buck, is modest, is humble, and doesn't crave the limelight. You will often find it working hard, behind the scenes. Even its very own name belies its greatness so that only those who understand its true worth ever seek out this diamond in the rough. That word is *health*. Its beauty is in its simplicity and in its raw naturalness, unadulterated and pure.

I know we've talked quite a bit about Isaiah 58:8, and its important yet again that we bring it back around for another new connection. If you recall, as a brief refresher: this is where Isaiah talks about fasting to break the bands of oppression and the wrong habits and things that bind us down to a type of slavery. He shares how we should use the food (or the funds we *would* have used to buy that food we would have eaten) to help feed the hungry. He says we should bring the poor into our homes and clothe the naked. In verse 8, he shares with us that when we do these things, *then* our light will break forth like the morning and our health will spring forth speedily. It is in this verse, above, that *health* references the word *healing* specifically. (I love the way that word rolls off the tongue in English—*healing*—I love to say it slowly: h-e-a-l-i-n-g...)

There is what was known as a Messianic Psalm, or a song about or relating to health and its *healing* power. However, in this particular song, "saving health" is more in reference to the salvation, the saving aspects of health. I'd hum a few bars for you, but I don't know the tune. The words go like this:

God be merciful unto us, and bless us, and cause his face to shine upon us; Selah.

That thy way may be known upon earth, thy saving health among all nations.

Let the people praise thee, O God; let all the people praise thee.

Then shall the earth yield her increase, God our God shall bless us.

God shall bless us; and all the ends of the earth shall fear him.

In Acts 27 [31] the word *health* references *safety*. Now why would the word *health* mean *safety*? you might wonder. To give a little context here, Paul was a prisoner at the time being transported by boat to Julius, one of Agustus's centurions. The travel was complicated by storms, great winds, and great peril. Paul advised that the sailors (and prisoners) to wait on an island before continuing the trip, but they didn't listen to him. To top it all off, they were at the very end of a fourteen-day fast.

The ship had come through a dangerous situation the night before where the sailors were sure it was going to crash on the rocks. So, they had thrown out four anchors to try and hold their spot until the sun came up so they could see how close to shore they were. This was so they could navigate in safely. However, Paul, being inspired, told the sailors that they needed to stay where they were in the boat but to pull up the anchors. If the men abandoned ship, they'd all drown. So, the sailors followed his direction, and everyone lived to see the next day.

As the sun rose, these sailors who had been straining between terrifying life and death experiences for weeks saw Paul coming through the dark of night with a loaf of bread. He begged them, imploring them to eat for their health.

(Okay maybe it was more than a single loaf. I hope so, or those would be just nibbles for each man. There were 276 souls onboard the ship!) All were given this meat, and it nourished them body and soul. This improved their moods, restored their strength and energy, and allowed them to continue their journey.

Food is a powerful resource, but if we are to enjoy long life and good health, more is required of us than to just eat. We have to actively take part in our own healing processes. The body's own natural ability to help balance, restore, and correct things and situations within it. However, I am *not* advocating bypassing necessary medical treatment.

Always work with your healthcare providers for advanced conditions. It is vital that you not misinterpret the writings in this book or mistakenly try to use it to diagnose, treat, or cure specific diseases. It is not intended for that purpose. This book is only for the purpose of strengthening and stabilizing general health in the body, mind, and spirit.

There was a good family who lived in Jerusalem who both the historical records mention and local people today still talk about. The family was very well known there and were very prosperous. The locals say they don't know where they disappeared to even to this day. One day they were there and the next they were just gone.

Unfortunately, they had to leave quickly because there were people in town who were plotting to murder them. The family escaped into the desert and traveled for some time. The sons in the family had quite a few squabbles over the decision to leave, over who was in charge, and where they were going. You know, basic sibling stuff.

Two of the sons were only interested in ruling the family according to the cultural traditions and having the power and the wealth. The other two sons were good and wise, like their parents. As the older sons began finding fault, living uncleanly, and sleeping longer than was needful, they began to pick on the other brothers more, repeatedly tearing them down. [46]

Instead of being drawn in to the fight by the two grumpy brothers (because he was more of an early to bed, early to rise kind of guy), one of the younger brothers reminded the older two about how grateful they should be and how much their ancestors, the Israelites who fled from Egypt, had sacrificed for them. He also reminded them of the healing event that had happened when the Israelites had hardened their hearts, just like the two older brothers were now doing. Then he reminded them that God had straightened out the Israelites when they got so out of line and off the plan.

God sent flying fiery serpents among the Israelites, who were bitten. Afterward, God prepared a way for the people to be healed. What they had to do was to *look*. Such a simple sounding thing, but when you think about it, it becomes apparent very quickly how scary and overwhelming looking *at* or even looking *into* something can become.

The excuses can come flying out, like, "I don't have time to look into that," or "I don't need to look at that, if it worked or was important someone else would tell me, so *I* don't need to do it," or "That just wouldn't work because ____" (fill in the blank with your tailored excuse of choice).

How often do we do this with nutrition? We blow it off because "it doesn't work" or "it doesn't affect anything." We don't have time. Even if it *was* true, X, Y, or Z agency would do A, B, C or make me do it. Or we say to ourselves, "I'll wait until later to look into it," and then we don't.

The way you were eating ten years ago has created the body you have and live in today. What you eat now is going to create the body you live in ten years from now. And in the Israelite camp, because *looking* was too easy, many people died. And people are *still* dying today because they refuse to do the simple things. You don't heal when you don't fuel.

Eventually these same four brothers became six brothers when the last two were born in the wilderness while the family wandered for physical safety and protection from those who would murder them. They tried to live the good laws of health. Soon enough, the two middle boys grew to be adults and one of them became the leader of their newly thriving community after their father passed away.

They had a special meeting and the older of the middle, good brothers wrote down what he said and also decided to share some of what Isaiah had written and compared this new group of people that was now their community to their ancestors. There is one particular part of this record that I find particularly striking because we know Isaiah primarily wrote about our last days that we live in now.

Isaiah had a vision where he saw God and became a bit panicked in front of God's glory, power, and purity. Realizing he was feeling undone and because he had unclean lips (because he lived among people of unclean lips) he was given a live coal to put on his lips to purge away his imperfections. When God asked for someone to go and prophesy to the people for him, Isaiah stepped up and said,

"Send me."

God told Isaiah to share a message with us, and this is what Isaiah wrote to us:

"Hear indeed, but they understood not, and see indeed, but they perceived not."

I think this happens a lot: we think we hear but we don't understand and believe we see but don't truly perceive. I think this happens especially if and when we are not in the habit of actively listening all the time. How often do we look right at something without really seeing it? This happened to me the other day. I was scrambling around looking for something, and I was in a hurry too. I couldn't find it, but it was right in front of me the whole time; I didn't see it until it was pointed out to me. We laughed about it, but only moments before I was frustrated and overwhelmed with worry. Things can be right in front of our faces, and we don't see what's so obvious. God continued:

"Make the heart of this people fat, and make their ears heavy, and shut their eyes; lest they see with their eyes, and hear with their ears, and understand with their heart, and be converted and be healed." [31]

Isaiah asked, "How long?" And God said, "Until the cities be wasted without habitation, and the houses without man, and the land be utterly desolate, And the Lord have removed men far away, and there shall be a great forsaking in the midst of the land. Only a very small percentage shall return and sprout back up."

Are our hearts so fat and heavy that we cannot understand the power of nutrition and the healing power of foods? Have our eyes been so shut tightly that we cannot see truth in front of us anymore? Have our ears closed off from hearing right principles? We cannot be converted to healthy eating or be healed if we cannot *look*. If we convert ourselves, God has promised to heal us. The message can't get through congested micro-organisms easily, though, so if he tells us—even if *I* tell you too—can you act and make the decision to get clear enough to receive the very important memo? The memo has been sent!

After the father's death, the next leader of the family community that had left Jerusalem, Jacob, was tasked with teaching proper principles for good health and living rightly before God, and he took that charge very seriously. He wished that he could persuade all the people to eat right and follow the laws given to make mankind happy and free. His compassionate heart gave him strength and courage to follow through.

No matter how much we are able to see with our own eyes, hear with our own ears, and understand with our own hearts, we can only do so much. Our effort, no matter how great or small, will only get us so far by our own merits. It is literally impossible for us to heal ourselves on our own. After we have done everything that we can do (impossible on our own), the difference still has to be made up by someone else who can. Because of our ancestors' choices (over which we had no control) and our own flaws and imperfections, a price must be paid to reclaim and recover us from the cry for justice to the right way.

This is where "the arm of the Lord is revealed" to us. God "was wounded for our transgressions." A *transgression* is the violation of a law, principle, or duty. It is a breach of contract. It means you've gone out of bounds. He was literally and figuratively bruised for our morally objectionable behavior and our unjust acts. "The chastisement of our peace was upon him," which means that we may have the opportunity to get peace in our lives again through living by God's laws.

With our Savior's stripes we are healed. He took the punishment for all the things we've done wrong, that for which no matter how long we perform restitution, we cannot repair what we've broken in ourselves or in someone else. Still, we are still required to valiantly attempt restoring back to good order what we've done wrong in an attempt to help others heal and forgive us, so we can forgive ourselves and receive forgiveness from those we have hurt, from God, and from ourselves.

It's not enough to just eat the right foods. We must also work through the mental and emotional traumas and spiritual issues involved with harmful eating habits, food abuse, and any other unhealthy and unwholesome practices. It's a process that cannot be done alone.

You need massage work, perhaps counseling, and nutritional support until you're strong enough to go on your own. This is not usually when you think you are ready for it. It takes quite a bit of time. Maybe you need support groups and spiritual counseling. Every situation is unique, and there is not one of us who hasn't needed help in one area or another.

Because of Christ, many of us may be justified but we have to choose it. We have to *choose* to eat good, healthy foods, to rest properly, to work and work to get better at it. Since the law was created, it requires the life of anyone who violates it because violating it because violating it is so offensive to God, especially in light of what is promised and given to us as a reward. Many ancient historical records *and* oral traditions across many religious belief systems point to the concept that we're here on earth and knowingly agreed to come be a part of this experience. We chose to go through all these things to learn about opposition and to prove ourselves. In exchange we can acquire contractual promises and blessings.

Since we cannot survive the high price of death and there being only one who was pure enough and blameless to pay it and survive, we are his and eternally indebted to him for this great sacrifice. But he loves us as his own bride and gives his life willingly on our behalf in order to restore us as before without blemish or blame.

What we eat is part of our covenant to be clean and pure before God. What we eat *matters*. It helps us fulfill the measure of our creation. *We* matter, so we should eat well and treat ourselves a healthier way. This is the birth of an upward healing spiral that will elevate and lift us higher. When we don't love ourselves, we tend to make worse food choices, and, likewise, poor eating habits can add to hating ourselves with each bite.

There was a man who happened to come across a group of people who were so down and out because they had been kicked out of their church for the simple reason that they were poor as to things of the world. It was a church that had become more and more wealthy over time, and those with great wealth began to look at the poor people in the church as nothing more than garbage that needed throwing out. This progressed to literally kicking those poor people to the curb. Worst of all were the priests, who treated the poor horribly and despised them.

When this man saw them so downhearted, he tried to lift their spirits and encourage them by pointing out that they could still worship even though they weren't part of a physical church. He pointed out that the poor had humbled themselves all this time on their own and chosen to have soft hearts—open hearts—without being forced to and how much better that was. He shared with them about nourishing the spiritual fruit on their tree of faith. Then, he reminded them of the many prophets who had come before them, including Moses, who spoke of the One who would come. Moses raised a symbolic representation of the brazen serpent when the Israelites were bitten by fiery flying serpents.

The brass serpent, a type, was raised and *all* the people had to do was *look* at it. Many did look, and they lived, but there were many people whose hearts were hardened and they were prideful. Many of the Israelites were so hardened they *refused* to look, and they died. Why didn't they look? They didn't *believe* it would heal them!

Now the man asked a question to the poor who had been kicked out of their church. "If you could be healed just by casting your eyes about, wouldn't you look quickly? Or would you be hard hearted and filled with unbelief, or even lazy? Would you *not* look and then die? If you want to be hard-hearted, bad things will happen to you. If you'd rather be the soft-hearted, then *look around* and live."

Is food going to fix everything on its own? No. It's not supposed to. Its purpose is to nourish the physical body. When the physical body is fully and properly nourished on an ongoing basis, it prevents a lot of potential problems. We have to remember, though, we are not just a physical body here to have only a physical experience. We also are an emotional body, a mental body, and a spiritual body. We are also here to have emotional experiences, mental ones, and, yes, even spiritual too. We are *all* these things, like it or not.

It's not any different than saying I have a right arm and a left one, and a right leg and a left one. You may hate your right arm, but that doesn't change the fact that it is a part of your complete makeup. Sometimes one or more of these parts may become imbalanced, sickly, or injured, and we may feel hatred for that part—but it's still *there*, is still ours, and once healed and in balance with the rest, it's happy again and *whole*. We cannot ignore the spiritual nourishment because it also affects the whole. When we are not properly nourished on all sides, it creates holes, weak areas in our defenses. It makes us open to attacks, whether from bacteria or other forms of threat: spiritual, mental or emotional.

An improper diet—whether physical, emotional, or spiritual—creates division within the body and destroys its ability to have all parts working together, and the bodily defenses and borders strong against potential mutiny or hostile takeovers. Our mental diet affects the mind and our thoughts; our experiential diet (how we choose to act or react) affects our emotions; and our balance of light and dark in our minds and hearts affects the spirit.

Before Christ was crucified on the cross, there was a community of people who could not agree any longer on common ground. They couldn't live with each other anymore. None could live for the common good, and they disbanded into separate groups apart from each other. Consequently, they became weaker. They lost their peace. This didn't just happen collectively but also individually. Their minds became hard as their hearts, and their minds became blind not only to those around them but also to the growing darkness within themselves.

There was one man, who had led them before these groups had separated themselves into their own communities. He realized what was happening and started going among them that very year, trying to help everyone restore their balance. He was a man of great power and authority in this service and he ministered to them. Because of this and walking in the truth so boldly, many people became angry with him because he had more and greater power than they did.

234

The people could *not* believe this man's words, even though he had such great faith that angels were ministering to him daily. However, many people eventually were able to find their balance again because of his hard work in restoring them to the gospel principles of God's law of health.

Many people who had devils cast out of them and were healed of their sicknesses and infirmities said that they had been healed by the Spirit of God. These same people went out and did miracles among the rest of the people as well. I'm sure you know by now that food imbalances can contribute to sickness and infirmities physically—and spiritual devils can contribute to them too.

I know this may be a scary topic to many. I think it's one of those topics for which we either just want to bury our heads in the sand or close our eyes and plug our ears while saying loudly "Nah-Nah-Nah-Nah! I can't hear you!"—pretending it's not there, it's not real: out of sight, out of mind. Or we feel like if we just don't think about it, then it doesn't exist.

There is a whole band width of colors and light that our eyes cannot even register. Cats can see more of these other colors and light waves than humans can. And, while people may not be able to see all these same band widths of color in general, some are able to see more than most and some see less than most. Just like some people are tall and some are more vertically challenged, some are good at sports and others have a talent for the arts, some people are good at helping balance the body and nourish it physically, emotionally, and spiritually.

Wherever you fall on that food nourishing and balancing spectrum, you can become better at it—a little each day with practice. Like any muscle that is used regularly and with a concentrated effort, the more you do something, the more you can develop the skill. You can develop confidence and strength and increased ability to handle yourself and cope with every part of your daily living. You are more powerful in this arena over things—even things *unseen*—than you may know.

Among the people we know of as some of the Native American tribes in the North American continent, there is a story in their history in which a lot of bad things were being done by those running their government. They were destroying their country and the people living in it, to get gain for themselves, and there were many who left and removed themselves to other lands so they could live safely and in freedom. The rest stayed, and whether they did not or *could* not see the coming dangers, they were not prepared for the coming events and calamities. This was around the same time the previously mentioned man had gone out ministering to the people, trying to restore balance among them.

The people knew that a man had come among them to remind them of a prophecy of a time of great darkness that would come and last for three days in conjunction with the crucifixion of Christ. Despite many signs and wonders being fulfilled in their time, a lot of people began to doubt that it would ever happen. There were even big arguments about it: the people's disagreements went on for a couple of years prior to this great darkness, so you can imagine the level of fights going on.

Then, there came a storm, a storm such that had never been seen before throughout *all* the land. The thunder alone was so loud, it shook the ground with enough force people thought it was going to split the earth in two. The lightning was so sharp, it was as though no one had seen or heard of it before. An entire city sank into the sea, and everyone in it drowned. Another city caught on fire.

A third city was completely covered with earth and turned into a giant mountain.

The whole southern part of their land experienced a terrible destruction. The entire face of the land was changed due to the thousands of earthquakes that happened. All their highways were completely broken up and destroyed. Everything smooth became rough and spoiled.

Poor nourishment can have a similar effect on the body: it can lead the body, mind, and spirit to be much more susceptible to a cataclysmic event that could potentially devastate and destroy, things like cancer, mental illness, and more.

There are many cultures that have a similar story in their cultures of a great God coming to visit them. These stories are found all around the world. This God who had healing power—in his touch, in his work. This is a theme you see repeated over and over, no matter where these stories are told. He came and he healed them. He loved them. And, they felt of his love for them, and *they loved him.*

The God that came to visit the people of the Americas in the days after the crucifixion of Jehovah (Jesus Christ, Jeshuah) in Jerusalem came after three days of intense darkness, earthquakes, and storms mentioned previously.
238

When he came, he showed them the prints in his hands and feet, he taught them, he prayed for them and blessed them.

As he finished teaching them, he told them he needed to return to *his* father. As he looked at them, he could tell that they did not understand everything he had come to tell them. So, he said they should go home, think about all the things he'd told them and return in the morning. He'd come back and give them more. When he looked at them again, he saw their eyes filled with tears and knew they wanted to ask him (without actually asking him) to stay longer with them.

He had so much compassion and mercy for them, and he said that he knew they wished he'd show and do to them what he did for those in Jerusalem. They believed and were ready to act on their belief—*that's* faith! The *power* to act. So, he told them he could see their faith was strong enough that he could heal them.

Then the most beautiful thing happened when the Great Peacemaker finished speaking. The people moved in unison and began to bring up to him all of the people who were sick, the blind, those with various afflictions, those who were lame, and those who couldn't speak. They brought everyone, and as they did, he healed them.

Can you imagine watching *this scene* unfold before your eyes? Can you *imagine* it?

They'd heard the stories and read the records saying he would come, how he'd come, and when. These were kept as oral and written records and handed down and protected carefully for many generations as a way of maintaining hope in those last days awaiting God's Son's arrival. They received a witness, a personal experience of healing, and their records are to give *us* hope so we can believe them as they testify of what they felt, saw, heard, and experienced. Timing is *everything*, as are life lessons.

Things don't always get handed to you in life. Sometimes—maybe even most times—we have to do our part; we have to work to get things. Nothing is free. And, when something is broken, *really* broken, it needs to be fixed or repaired so it can be restored to new again.

As an example: if a wall or even a bone gets a crack in it, it needs to be recreated first as a state of spirit matter and then in the physical. There should be a planning process to determine the best course of action. We need to diagnose the situation and figure out how extensive the damage is, what supplies are needed, and if more items need to be acquired.

What resources do we already have on hand, and which need to be collected? Where do we need to go to get the materials, and is that something that can be sourced locally or is it something that needs to be bought and shipped first? Will this be a simple project that we can do ourselves, or "DIY" it, or is this going to require additional hands or someone with more knowledge or expertise to make the repair? These are all important considerations. Also, how will we handle and deal with the emotional fallout or fears associated with the healing process?

When the Great Peacemaker returned the next morning as he had promised the Native American people, he gave them some mandates to help them renew and restore themselves and help strengthen each other because some were not ready to go through the complete and deep healing process. We are not allowed to dictate someone else's process or timing, but we are required to be there, to give them support, and show them love. We are to continue to minister to those who are not yet ready because we do not know if or when they might *become* ready to be healed. When they *are* ready for it, he will heal them. Jesus told the Native Americans during that time to be the means of helping bring this salvation to those individuals among them, when they were ready.

The Great Peacemaker is all about restoring things that are broken. That is why he has come and given us God's laws of health and nutrition, so we can nourish our physical bodies. When we eat right, our bodies, minds, and spirits can start to work the way they are supposed to. And, when things work the right way, we feel better, we can do better, and we can live better lives filled with more joy and happiness.

When trials and difficulty come into our lives— and they will—we can handle them better and with more grace and thanksgiving. We start to have the ability to focus on healing the mind, the heart, and the soul. *That's* when things really start to get exciting in our lives. Yes, I just said *start* twice in a row, and it was intentional because" it's time. To. Start.

We only have today, this moment. That conviction you are feeling right now is the spirit confirming to you that you need to engage yourself—*now*. Take your foot off the brake pedal, take yourself out of park, and *drive.* All it takes is a little bit of faith. Your destination awaits!

Combine your power to act on things you cannot yet see—faith—with your belief that God is all powerful, able, and willing. When we align our hearts and our minds with his will, he has promised us that he will do miracles, signs, and wonders to all those who believe in his name. Don't get impatient, now, and try to skip steps and jump to the end! You still have to follow the rules like the laws of nature, physics, gravity, and more; just like God does.

Good things only come after a trial of our faith. That means there's going to be a testing period that you have to complete to show that you really mean it, are doing it for the right reasons, and are going to keep enduring and following through. Don't go wastin' miracles! Do the work. Be real. Be authentic. Get the results.

When we fulfill the required obligations that demonstrate our belief in God and we ask for it in his name, he has promised us that we can—and in fact *shall*—cast out devils. Remember some of those addictions you've been unsuccessfully struggling to break free of (food or otherwise)? That's right: Cast. Them. Out! Belief is the key; use the power and authority of God's name to do it.

God also promised that you shall heal the sick. Did you know that around 94% to 96% of natural illnesses have an emotional or spiritual root cause? That sounds really high, right? Initially, I thought the same thing. I am skeptical and I *do* filter ideas before I let them continue their way through my brain. Not only was the researched information there before my eyes (and it was convincing), it still had to pass my rigorous self-test phase. So, I did it. I tested it on myself. Once I was convinced, I tested it out on those willing participants around me next, and it held up again. It didn't even flinch or bat an eye. My curiosity become hope, and my hope turned to knowledge. With years of practice, my knowledge became wisdom.

We were also promised that those who believe, and ask in his name shall cause the blind to receive their sight and the deaf to hear. Not only did the Great Peacemaker's disciples do this, but even some people who were not in their church were doing it. It's not a "holier than thou" thing or a "this person has more power or authority" thing. It's an "obey the laws and the good consequences follow" thing. Do the work, follow the rules for the results you want to achieve, and see the results. The dumb shall speak, and the lame will walk.

In reference to the Law of Health that we've been given, there is a contingency, a possibility for which we can prepare but when we're not sure what will happen. This is for those who have *no* faith to be healed, but *still* believe.

This is God's Law, God's contingency. I'm just sharing the information. It says, that for all those who believe, but have not faith to be healed, they should be nourished with herbs and mild food with all tenderness and not by the hand of the enemy for their physical health's sake. [56] Now, why is this? Your body can't do what it needs without proper energy and resources. As we've already mentioned, the body needs variety, it needs balance, it needs whatever is missing!

We've discussed foods cooked and raw, and we've talked about fruits and vegetables. The use of herbs and mild foods are also very healing for our bodies. These types of food have power. Something very important that is included in this law is that the people who are ill are *not* to be nourished or given any of these things by the hands of an enemy.

Now this last part is very easily brushed off and far too often dismissed and ignored. There are implications and indicators, however, that it's happening way more than we'd like to think—and in ways that we couldn't have even imagined. A person who is not well needs *more* protection from enemies because they usually are not able (or, at least, less able) to protect themselves.

Before you go and beat yourself up: even if you've asked God to heal you but you weren't immediately healed, don't think this necessarily means that you're evil, hopeless, or forgotten. There are *many* reasons why people are not instantly healed by faith. Sometimes it is part of a trial of our faith before we receive the blessing. Will you keep trying, working towards the right way, even if you haven't gotten there yet? Or will you quit just as soon as you gain your reward? Sometimes we're ready now, and sometimes there are other factors at play. Usually, the other factors are things that we don't even realize.

Not everyone is good at the same things. Some people are really good at cooking or baking. Others are good at growing foods and plants. Still others are good at teaching. These are gifts given to those individuals for the benefit of those who love God and keep all his laws and those who are trying to do so. It is done this way so that anyone that seeks him or ask him for healing (not for a sign for their own lusts) can later share so that all may benefit for good. Some are given one gift, and others are given many.

A gift is different than a talent. A talent is something that you develop, practice, or repeat until you are accomplished at it. A talent is something for which you may have a natural knack. It's something that comes easily and naturally to you. A gift is something that just *is* already there. One of those gifts might be "given to have faith to be healed." To others they might have the faith to heal other people. So, you may (or may not) have the gift to be healed by faith. That's not a defect one way or another. Whatever gifts we *do* have are meant to be a blessing to *others*.

What about bishops, pastors, apostles, and prophets? Are they faultless or called to their positions because they're more holy, wise, or above temptation? Those called to positions of authority or leadership are *not* exempt from answering to all the same laws and requirements that you and I are. There is *more* accountability, not less. Not only do they have to answer for their own choices and mistakes, but they have a greater responsibility for those over whom they have stewardship.

The Great Spirit made an admonition regarding how to best stay in "the way" when it comes to our leaders. The words we speak will feel like a rebuke to those not following the right laws as set forth by the Lord, he says. We are to be humble when doing this, relying on God to lead us in what to say and when; we are to pray for guidance. Similarly, we are not to exalt our leaders nor to love them about other people (an easy trap many fall into); we should only love them as ourselves and as all other men, the same as those who love God.

We must pray for our leaders—in the church *and* in the government—to make good, wise laws and choices. And, when they make mistakes, we *are* to admonish them sharply to be faithful to God first and foremost. This is *not* a task we can leave to others; it comes down squarely on each of our shoulders, and we have a responsibility to do it *and* answer to God for doing it or not. Either way, we are accountable as well.

Our church and government leaders will be held accountable by God. After their trials and temptations, and lots of tribulation, God will feel out their true hearts to see if they've softened or hardened them and grown stubborn and rebellious to change. If these leaders have not stiffened their necks and stayed bristled against good, healthy connection, will be converted, and change their wayward ways, then he will heal them. [58] Leaders, are more responsible, but we all have to answer for our part. That's what makes society great for everyone, not just the majority and not only for the leaders: for *everyone* participating. If

248

we *all* lift each other up, we will have a society that benefits every single member of the community.

We are all so different, and the things we *do* need to cover everyone requires balance and variety, just like our nutritional diets. "One-size-fits-all" never works for everyone, and it's a bit dishonest if you think about it. Have you ever tried wearing a one-size-fits-all shirt before? While some absolutely swim in fabric, the shirt is way too tight for others. Still others can't even get their head through the neck hole (let alone the rest of themselves), and others could sink into the neck opening and crawl in and out of it.

We must hold everyone to the same high standards: those with power over our food must be held to the standard of the ones who created the plants, the animals, and the earth; and those who handed down the laws to govern them all and rule them. Anything else, tries to create a one-size-fits-all world and history has repeatedly shown that a one-size-fits-all world just doesn't work.

Everything that grows and flourishes follows certain laws, rules, and ordinances. We must follow them too if we want to thrive. If we seek for nourishment—*true* nourishment, not just the outward appearance of it—we will be rewarded. All followers of the Great Peacemaker "who remember to keep and do [the things we've discussed in this book], will receive health in their navel and marrow in their bones."

Read that again: you will "receive health in [your] navel and marrow in [your] bones." Why is this significant from a nutrition standpoint? Well, if you had a well from which to draw water, wouldn't you want there to be water in it?

As it relates to our health metaphorically, nutrition is the bucket that enables us to draw the life-giving water from the well and the rain that refills the well with water again. Without nutrition, we cannot accomplish what we need to accomplish in this life. We *must* have it in order to access and even to maximize the potential of our wellness. You might be wondering, why does this even matter?

Throughout my life, I have thought that I felt pretty good. In fact, I have felt downright healthy and vibrant (for what I thought "healthy" was) most of my life growing up. Sure, I had regular colds, and bumps and scrapes, and even a few surgeries and surprises, but who doesn't on some level expect that? You may have higher or lower expectations for yourself than I did for myself. I realize that.

I make allowances for that in my pondering of what would be most useful for each one of you to know.

What I came to realize for myself was I could not entirely know *myself* the way I thought I could or did. It has only been as I have gone along my own wellness journey, seeking "The Way" and doing my best with incomplete knowledge, that I have only *begun* to see with my own eyes and to hear with my own ears, metaphorically speaking.

We each can only journey as fast and as far as we are able. There is an amazing journey waiting for you in nutrition, I promise. You may not realize it now, but once you're on the other side of it, you may find it has been one of the most fantastic journeys of your life!

This historical story about a religious leader applies perfectly as an analogy to our own human bodies and the many purposes it serves for us. So, think about this story in relation to that.

There was a group of men—about four of them, if I recall correctly—who received inspiration from God to build a house in the community where they resided. The house had multiple purposes. The first was that the house needed to serve as a boarding house. It would be a place for strangers from near and far to lodge there. Second, it needed to be a good house, worthy of acceptance by all who came to stay there; it needed to be a place where weary travelers would find health and safety. The house needed these things so that those who stayed there could comfortably contemplate the word of God while they were there, as well as the cornerstone that he had appointed for Zion. Third, it was to be built in God's name and intended as a *healthful* habitation: It was to not have *any* pollution to come *in* it or *upon* it (so that it would be holy).

I get *so* happy thinking about visiting such a place and dwelling there for a visit before passing through. Imagine walking into such a place. It's clean, and it's got this wonderful natural sunlight streaming in through the windows. You see a table spread with freshly prepared foods being set for you as you walk in. It sounds like heaven to me!

If it truly *was* heaven, or even the Garden of Eden, which was reputedly a literal paradise, what sorts of nourishing foods would we see on that table? More than likely there might be a variety of herb-bearing seeds, fruits from every tree, and dishes made from all types of plants and herbs. These foods were given to our first father and mother, and to all the animals, to eat. I wonder what fruits taste like where the soil is so rich and full of nutrients and plants produce their seed spontaneously. [32]

Imagine walking up to a tree and plucking off a perfectly ripe fruit without any toiling required to maintain the tree; it might be the most delicious thing you ever tasted. We know that things were not allowed to stay in such a state. Unfortunately, Adam and Eve made choices that got them expelled from the garden. Thus began their life of hard work, weeding and living by the sweat of their brows, as they say.

Time passed, and a lot of things happened, and the earth changed. Adam and Eve had quite a few children. Generations passed; Noah (of the great flood) was part of the 10th generation, counting Adam and Eve as the first.

After the flood, Noah and his family were able to depart the boat, called an *ark* in the Bible. They were given a blessing from God, who told them that he had put fear and dread of mankind into all the animals, fowls, and fishes. Every *living* thing that *moved* would be food for Noah and his descendants, which includes all of us. Likewise, every green herb will be given for his and our use. [33] However, God was very specific about also telling the people, from Noah on, *not* to eat the *blood* of the animals.

The blood should be shed *upon* the ground, which takes the life. The guideline given for taking the life of an animal is that it should only be taken and used for meat to save your own life. For each animal's life we take, we will have to account to God for.

Similarly, human blood is equally precious to God, and he said we are not to shed another human's blood; the punishment for *murder* is that the murderer's *blood* must be *shed* by man to make payment and restitution for his or her crime. There is no other acceptable way given. Everyone should strive to preserve the life of mankind. And, like the Garden of Eden, like our first parents, we are to seek to multiply and replenish the earth abundantly. [34]

We know that we don't have the whole story, but we do the best we can with the parts of the story that we *do* have. We must be careful in how we are to handle and manage the resources we have available to us. It starts with our food and then ripples out to plants and animals on the planet.

Eating the right way can give us hope. Eating the *wrong* way can contribute to feelings of despair and despondency. Food can throw off a body's hormone levels, or it can help rebalance them. This is part of the reason it is so important to observe moderation in all things. We must practice self-control and—in certain situations and under some conditions—abstinence.

Now a perfect and terrifying example of misuse of ceremonial foods comes to us from the days and times of Moses of Egypt. This is the same Moses who freed a portion of the Israelites from the slavery under the Pharaoh. Moses had an older biological brother named Aaron, and Aaron had two sons: Nadab and Abihu.

These two sons were a part of the generation who had been delivered from Egypt, so they'd been slaves their whole lives, they wandered in the desert, and they had seen and experienced quite a few miracles along the way. Nadab and Abihu had been selected to be part of a group made up of Moses, Aaron and an additional seventy elders. The group gathered and had the opportunity to eat before God and worship from afar while Moses and his minister, Joshua, went up to Mount Sinai to meet with God and get the stone tablets with the statements and laws inscribed on them. Moses went closer to talk with the Lord and returned to report what God had said (along with God's judgments).

Now, fast forward a little, the Israelites constructed a tabernacle, as they'd been commanded to do, and Aaron and his sons had been washed, anointed, and given the everlasting priesthood. They were trained in all of the ceremonial sacrifices that must be made on behalf of the people, and finally the day came when Aaron made the first sacrifice. Everything was done as God commanded, and God accepted this pure offering by burning it up with fire.

To really appreciate the situation and understand what happened, remember that Aaron and his sons (and the other men) had gone through a seven-day long purification ceremony. They did this so that they would be clean and found worthy before the Lord while working in the tabernacle and making acceptable sacrifices before him. At some point, though, after Aaron's sacrifice (which had been done correctly), Nadab and Abihu got drunk and went in with incense on their own and "offered a strange fire" which was an inappropriate offering.

God has said that any form of disobedience cannot exist in God's presence, so when they made this unholy offering (that they had been warned not to do or they would die), the two men were burned up and killed (instead of burning up the sacrifice, as he had done with Aaron before). [64] God had *Moses* tell Aaron that God would be sanctified in them that drew near to me, and that God will be glorified before all men. And Aaron, being humbled, held his peace.

So, then Moses grabbed a couple of his nephews, the sons of Uzziel, and had them remove the two burned bodies from the tabernacle and take them clear outside of the camp. They followed very specific instructions from God so they themselves would not die.

After that, God spoke to Aaron and told him: no wine at all nor fermented drinks when going to the tabernacle of the congregation or you may die too. God acknowledged that this was a new rule, but it was to be done so that it would be very easy to tell the difference between what is holy and what is not, between what was clean and what was unclean.

We should *also* take care what we put into our bodies for similar reasons. (Not that we are going to be priests entering a temple to offer up sacrifices to God the way Aaron and his sons were.) However, the cleaner we are on the inside, the more access we have to peace, harmony, and enlightenment within our own selves. We will be stronger and happier and feel safer too.

Let's talk about what a Nazir Vow is for a moment. Have you heard of it? I hadn't realized how heavily prevalent it was during Bible times. So common was the practice (during the time of the Old Testament) that they didn't really mention it so much in the records we carry around with us in the Bible.

According to the Mishnah, the first written collection of Jewish oral traditions, also called the Oral Torah, there was a queen by the name of Queen Helena of Adiabene. (This would have been circa 48 CE.) She placed herself under a Nazarite Vow for seven years on the condition that her son returned home from war safely.

Once Queen Helena's son returned home safely from the war, as was her condition for taking the Vow upon herself, she began fulfilling her end of the covenant: a seven-year-long commitment of purification. At the end of seven years, she headed to Jerusalem and took with her the required animals and offerings to sacrifice there. However, when she arrived, members of the School of Hillel told her that she needed to redo it. So, she did.

When Helena was almost finished with this second attempt, she became ritually impure by corpse uncleanness, and this caused her vow to become null and void. So, she started over a third time: a seven-year process from the beginning. Finally, after twenty-one years she completed her seven-year vow. (Not all Nazir Vows are seven years long. It can be for any set amount of time or it can be for a lifetime.)

When a Nazir Vow is taken, the Nazarite is required to do the following:

1. Abstain from wine and all grape products such as vinegar, grapes, raisins, etc.
2. Refrain from cutting the hair on their head.
3. Avoid ritual impurity by touching or contacting corpses or graves, even those of family members

After meeting the requirements for the set amount of time specified in the person's vow, the Nazarite offers a specific animal sacrifice and the Nazarite's hair is shorn off and burned. They are described as being "holy" and "holy unto God" but at the same time have to bring a sin offering. The word *Nazarite* means "consecrated, separated."

Foods are used to make promises. For the Nazier Vow, these offerings are: an unblemished lamb as a burnt offering, an ewe as a sin offering, and a ram as a peace offering. (Additionally, three more offerings accompany the peace offering: a basket of unleavened bread, a grain offering, and a drink offering.)

God said to Moses that when someone (man or a woman) decides to separate themselves unto the Lord and vow the vow of a Nazarite, they should not drink wine or strong drink—alcoholic beverages. They should not drink vinegar wine or vinegar of strong drink, and they should not drink any grape juice, or eat grapes, or raisins. [35]

We have to separate ourselves; just like the Nazarites separated themselves in their vows to God, we must *also* choose to separate ourselves from the foods that harm us.

God told the Israelites who separated themselves from Egypt that if they were to be holy (the opposite of common or profane) if they would be unique peculiar—and chosen—they should not eat anything that was abominable, heathenistic, loathsome, or of immoral practice. [36]

What is *common* is going to look like? It means to go along with what the crowd's doing—being and doing the easy thing, what the world calls "cool," "hot," or "phat." Look around; it's likely going viral on the internet. It may appear good on the surface, but if you test it out, it will prove itself to be darkness and destruction on the inside. It will consume you and throw you out like yesterday's news.

These things destroy whereas, the laws of nutrition bring us health to our navels. [37]

Did you know that the navel is a central part of anything, even the body? It is a port entrance for nourishment.

In the womb, we each obtained this nourishment from our mother through the blood vessels of the umbilical cord, from which we received other life-sustaining functions as well. When we consume and bring the ways of the world into our bodies, we are slowly destroyed, rotting from the inside out. We don't see or feel the effects for a long time, but this method is the most destructive of all; you can't stop something you can't see coming. Once you begin to see the rot on the outside, it's already too late.

You metaphorically go in to operate, and everything inside is already black and died long ago. Now it may be unrevivable and not enough good left for you to salvage anything.

Herein lies the danger. If we only concern ourselves with the upkeep of our external bodies, we miss the roles, duties, and responsibilities to honor, sacrifice, and receive the rewards from our daily offerings. If you struggle to eat right and make good nourishment choices, the internal rot has already begun and must be reversed *immediately* before further damage occurs.

How this damage has come about matters in determining the best ways to restore those places within you and support making different choices and continuing on the path to wellness. This is why this is not something that should be done alone.

We cannot see ourselves clearly nor even fully trust all our experiences and perceptions, and we cannot support nor motivate ourselves when we're down and out, wanting to quit, or go grab that donut. How we find our way out of lifelong learned habits and belief systems, likewise, cannot be overturned in one day either. What we eat affects our blood. What we *don't* eat *also* affects the blood. Everything comes back to water—and to blood.

Blood carries the nutrients we need to survive to our body parts, and it hauls off the waste things that we no longer need, and what no longer works. When we eat right, we receive "marrow to [our] bones." Physically, bone marrow is the soft fatty tissue inside of our bone cavities. It forms components of the blood, including red and white blood cells as well as platelets. Bone marrow *must* be healthy in all three aspects of the wellness triangle so that we continue to survive.

Bone marrow conditions may have the following symptoms:

- Bleeding easily
- Bruising
- Fatigue
- Frequent infections
- Muscle weakness

How much more impact could you have upon your own body by just giving extra thought to what you're eating to nourish the marrow in *your* bones? Support the parts of your body that your bone marrow produces: the blood, muscles, and bones. Eat healthy.

They say that wine is a mocker. It treats the body, mind, and spirit with contempt. If a *person* was openly showing you disdain or raging against you verbally or even physically, would you just put up with it? [38] Likely not. So why would we do any less when it comes to how *foods* treat us?

I know I'm throwing down some hard-to-digest thoughts here. If you need to let it cook-down a bit and soften up some for easier assimilation, go for it. Just make sure to keep making those little advancements. Baby steps. We *cannot* allow ourselves to keep fooling ourselves; things have *changed.* Foods *affect* us; *nourishment* affects us. It matters; it *definitely* makes a difference.

Perhaps, when we were children, we learned to use food as a crutch to meet our neglected needs and to compensate for losses and shortages in life: the unmet need to be loved or not feeling worthy in general. Maybe we have or are still punishing ourselves with it. Perhaps we've used food to help us deal with overwhelming stress and to fill the empty void of despair, loneliness, and boredom. Poor eating choices and food abuse can quickly become an insatiable secret love affair, and our appetites can grow. As these appetites grow—sometimes without our even noticing— they may quickly become uncontrollable; our self-control becomes weaker due to lack of use and may even become paralyzed. But is this entirely *true? Will* we no longer have any self-discipline?

If you are to dine with a ruler, very carefully consider what foods are placed in front of you. If you are a person who is prone to appetites, put a metaphorical knife to your own throat and do *not* partake of the delicacies placed in front of you. [39] *That* food is deceitful. The ruler seems like they're *for* you (on your side) by offering these to you, but his heart is not with you. What you eat up, you will regret and vomit up later. Those foods will not be sweet anymore. When we overindulge—whether with wine or foods, it creates situations of poverty. [40]

Symptoms of overindulgence may include:

- Monetary poverty
- Emotional poverty
- Psychological poverty
- Drowsiness
- Dressing in rags or even wearing things you can't actually afford to be wearing, trying to look the opposite but overcompensating

Overindulging in relation to monetary poverty is about focusing excessively on or prioritizing remedying financial poverty. This happens often at the expense of addressing other important aspects in connection with poverty. Some of these other considerations that need to come first financially are things like food, shelter, clothing, and other goods that are normally obtained through purchases in the marketplace. This does not mean things like our education, basic infrastructure, and healthcare are not included as a part of this. In order to alleviate this, we have to consider the root causes of the monetary poverty and clear this up directly. No one else and no other way will truly help you reach your destination out of financial poverty other than addressing the root causes rather than chasing the symptoms of it, as many people tend to focus on.

Some ways we can begin addressing our monetary poverty is to take a balanced approach between monetary and non-monetary lack in our lives. We can invest in education, whether that's self-education, learning a trade, or going to college. Another thing we can look to is making sure we have basic infrastructures in place and how we can access various types and methods of healthcare. [41] Tracking our progress as we go along helps us not only keep track of where we are on the journey but also be able to increase our ability as we go. Finally, we can also research ways to change our situation in ways that will honor and elevate us and increase our true self-esteem.

Having underdeveloped or neglected emotional intelligence is a form or emotional poverty. This can lead a person do having difficulties in recognizing, regulating, and understanding their emotions and those of other people's.

The opposite of this would be to address it and overcome it. Some consequences of overindulging in emotional poverty are things like experiencing increased stress and anxiety—chronically so, not just over an occasional situation—people struggle to cope with the emotions they feel and their relationships with others. They often struggle with poor emotional regulation making it challenging to manage their emotions which can lead to irritability, impulsive behaviors, and mood swings. There is an inability to recognize and respond to others' emotions which can damage relationships due to a lack of ability to empathize and communicate effectively. Mental health issues like increased risk of mental health disorders like depression, anxiety disorders, and personality disorders are increasingly an issue. Overindulging in emotional poverty can make it harder to form healthy, fulfilling relationships, may hinder personal growth, and can stifle emotional intelligence development.

Factors that may contribute to overindulging in emotional poverty are things like a lack of emotional validation. This would be things like inconsistent or absent emotional validation from our caregivers or even our friends, those we date, or are married to. Things like how much and what type of exposure we have to abuse, chronic stress, or trauma can create a disruption in our healthy development in this area. We can also see the consequences from things like a lack of resources and social isolation. This can also include the forced suppression of emotions or making people prioritize logic over emotions.

Ways we can work on breaking the cycle of overindulgence in emotional poverty are by doing things like making self-care a top priority in your life; eating healthy, stretching and exercise, mindfulness and meditation, promoting emotional well-being and resilience. Surround yourself with people who validate and support you emotionally and helping you feel safe and understood and allowing you to do the same for them. Going to therapy and joining support groups can also help you discover and address things you didn't realize were an issue and finding better ways to cope emotionally. Another thing you can do is to learn as much as you can about empathy, self-awareness, and effective ways of communicating. One of the first and most important things to do to start becoming more emotionally rich is to recognize and acknowledge your emotions, good or bad. They are just emotions. What matters is what you do with them and that determines the good and bad of it. Suppressing or denying them makes us go emotionally bankrupt and we don't have to go there.

Psychological poverty may shock you a bit. When people are distracted during activities that are enjoyable—eating, socializing, taking a break—they can experience reduced satisfaction. This leads to overcompensation and overconsumption of pleasurable activities later. There can also be reduction of confidence in your ability to succeed, and short-sighted decision-making.

Overindulgence is known as being an excessive, indulgent behavior often accompanied by a lack of self-control or moderation, wasting limited resources or overspending. In this case, drowsiness is a symptom of the emotional and mental exhaustion that accompanies overindulgence. It doesn't matter whether you're spending money, time, or resources, the spending is happening and then what you've spent is gone. The feelings that follow are things like hopelessness, despair, and disempowerment. Overindulging is a form of self-destruction which creates more poverty and reduces chances of escaping or improving your situation and drowsiness will clothe a man in rags.

Not only does dressing in rags not look good, it also signals to others a lack of self-control by the wearer of the raggy clothing. You will lose out on opportunities that might have otherwise come to you and people may flat out avoid you, or you may attract the wrong type of attention. These things correlate directly to how we eat, how we feed and nourish the body. If you eat *incorrectly,* you will attract the wrong things and lose out on opportunities that you might have otherwise had.

The wise King Solomon said a land is blessed when its leader is the son of strength and its rulers eat at the right times of the day and year. They don't just laze around glutting themselves on fine foods all day long, neglecting their work and responsibilities. They are wise, not irresponsible of their duties; they use wisdom and order in all things. They eat only to give themselves strength, and not for literal or metaphorical drunkenness. [41] If this holds true for the leaders of lands, is this not also true for the rulers (so to speak) of our bodies as well? A king must come from the people, and the people support, follow, defend, and protect the land. Is this not true, then, for our bodies following, defending, and protecting our*selves?*

One cell that's healthy and strong cannot continue on and lead a body that is sick. It can only command a body that is in alignment with itself. If we want to be healthy, mustn't we be in line with the full functioning requirements needed to maintain a healthy immune system for defense of our bodies' borders? We must eat at the right times. We must regularly and consistently sleep early and early in the nighttime if we are to be wise, if we are to keep our brains and our guts healthy.

Let us strengthen our bodies—the muscles and our organs. It is just as much a battle to fight for good health; it requires strategy and cunning as much as a game of chess, Stratego, or checkers does. You are fighting—both literally and metaphorically—for your life!

When we don't make things the right way, like the foods we eat and the liquids we drink, we will experience undesirable consequences. It doesn't matter if we realize it or not; we are not going to be allowed the ignorance card from the Law of Cause and Effect. God requires us to educate ourselves as much as we can in this life about as much as possible.

Can't afford a college education? All those same college books are accessible and available through the library! You won't have the fancy paper saying you know all that stuff, but you will know all that stuff, and that's the important part. (I'm not so sure college and university diplomas really mean so much anymore with all the rumors of corruption and giving out honorary degrees to people who never did the work to earn them. They don't mean so much when there's so many people lying and cheating to say they got them but not really doing the work to earn them, themselves.)

In reference to drinking wine: there's more than one way to get drunk. Sure, drunk on wine – there are plenty of people who are mighty in wine and those who mix their strength with fermented beverages. [42] God says that these people will be filled with as many woes as those who are drunk on power, slavery, and corruption in the days of the return of the Messiah to the earth.

As we go barreling towards that day when Christ returns, have we contemplated in our hearts, on our own bellies and appetites? What do we need to leave behind to lighten our toxic load as we walk along desolate roads? Apparently, we have a decision to make. Do we continue marching to the beat of the drum of a drummer who is leading us to who-knows-where, or do we slip into the quiet, narrow path that leads to light, hope, and happiness with each bite that we take?

Our choices affect everything, and someday you will have to choose between *morality* and *legality that's immoral.* You will have to decide to do what is right and wrong. That moment is *now*. That bite is *now*. That food consequence is already affecting you *now*.

You don't have time to wait. Our diets now affect us ten years down the road. It is said when Christ returns, the world will be in such a state of bad choices that everything will be desolate and in a cursed situation. Music will cease, joy and mirth will die, and none who drink wine will be in song. Those fermented drinks, likewise, will leave those who drink them bitter. [43]

Physical, emotional, spiritual: these are all types of things to come, and we must sort them out and overcome them. We have no need for things that will corrupt us. Instead: health. Health in our navel. Marrow in our bones. Strength. Internal power. Endurance. *These* are the things we naturally crave. Fake substitutes may temporarily fool our stomachs, but eventually the body and spirit catch on; they know the difference.

Bad foods and things we take into ourselves can only destroy, never build up. It is deception.

After Christ died on the cross, there fell a great apostacy on the earth. An apostacy from what, you ask? From truth, from a fullness of knowledge. Isaiah, a man whose writings and prophecies have gone misunderstood for thousands of years, was writing about times far distant from his time. He was writing about *our* days.

Isaiah spoke of a time when Christ will return a second time to a small remaining number of people as a crown of glory. That his spirit of judgment will sit for a strength to them that will turn the battle to the gate. The term "turn the battle to the gate" is a military phrase meaning to *repulse* an enemy and drive them, not just out of your own city, but to drive them out all the way back to *their* own city's gate and besiege them *there*.

If you have bad bacteria or whatever illness overrunning your body causing chaos and disorder to your systems, you have one of two choices:

A. Throw your hands up in the air, give up, and cry

B. Maybe cry first – there's no shame, then get organized, clean your metaphorical house, and start throwing out the bad stuff.

That's right: all those store-bought, branded cookies; the convenient, processed boxed foods in the pantry; the preservatives; the processed sugars and dyes. Get as natural as you can. Get back to basics. Eliminate the foods that feed inflammation and wage war on your good cells.

274

Isaiah warns us that those in the last days before Christ's return will err through wine and through fermented drinks and will be out of their way: "the priest and the prophet have erred through fermentation, swallowed up of wine... erring in vision, and do stumble in judgment.") [44]

We are all equally fallible, in other words. Because our bodies are susceptible to corruption, we must be vigilant in watching ourselves. We must be vigilant in watching ourselves. We must have the strength and conviction of Daniel. The king intended for a portion of his food from his own table to be set aside and used to feed these kidnapped children while they were trained for their new duties. That's a lot of pressure! But Daniel committed in his heart that he would not defile himself with the king's food or wine no matter what happened. Daniel asked the head eunuch not to have him do this. [45]

How many miracles occurred because Daniel was so committed to staying true to the laws of good health? *You* can accomplish miracles too! Your commitment muscle will get stronger the more you exercise it. On one side of the coin, we have been shown an example to follow to be a person of strong commitment to eating and drinking things that bring good health and balance to the body. Every coin has two sides; a head and a tail. Daniel is a good first example, so we'll out him on the head of the coin. On the tail side we have an example from a lesser-known, lower prophet also known as a teacher in the Old Testament named Habakkuk.

Based on his little, three-page book in the Bible, Habakkuk lived around 605 BC. There is very little known about him except that he was warning Jerusalem, like many others were at that time: the Babylonians were going to come in and destroy them if they didn't change their bad habits and choices. Based on what he wrote, it's clear he was foreseeing a lot of disturbing things. On the subject of wine, he gives a warning: "Woe unto him that giveth his neighbor drink, that puttest thy bottle to him, and makest him drunken also, that thou mayest look on his nakedness!" [46] In other words: to those who are giving and forcing someone else to drink and become drunk with the specific intention that they can look on their nakedness, bad things await those who participate in this behavior. Woe is a very harsh warning and a descriptive punishment of how that will feel.

Certain things spring instantly to my mind in our day today regarding alcohol. (I'm sure you're probably thinking of them too, and so I won't go more into detail.) The purpose of my writing is *not* to disturb you so much as to inform and let you decide to do further research, if you wish, or to take action, if that is your desire.

Forcing someone else to eat, drink, or take *anything* is not okay, and Habakkuk makes that very clear. He was right about Jerusalem being destroyed by Babylon (they didn't stop their self-destructive ways and were destroyed), and it's safe to say anything *else* he says is—at the very least—worth weighing and considering heavily.

If you recall, Paul—the tentmaker and apostle— reminded the saints in Christ's church while in Corinth that *they,* themselves, were temples. He said to them:

Don't you know that you are the temple of God, and that the spirit of God dwells within you? If anyone defiles the temple of God, God will destroy that person, for the temple of God is holy, which temple you are. [47]

Defile is Greek in origin and means "to spoil, corrupt, deprave." If refers to keeping cleanliness of body, mind, and spirit and removing and avoiding any type of filthiness so that the holy ghost (or, holy spirit) can communicate through you and warn you in times of danger. Defilement is a kind of pollution that can be external or internal, and God considers it a sacrilege and unclean.

The Hebrew origin of the word *defile* is "lawlessness," which I like even more. It seems to cover more ground in fewer words, for one. God has given a clear law about how we are to care for and treat our bodies. Anything that goes against that violates his law and creates chaos and disorder, and he is a God of order.

There is a big difference between order and control. The latter is created from a place of force, which violates God's law of agency. Order, however, is a set way to do things for the greatest happiness that someone can choose willingly. It is not micromanaging, which only creates a false sense of order. That falls under controlling (or trying to control) others; it never ends well.

God is very good about the letter of the law. It has its place. But he also does not neglect the *spirit* of the law along with it. One does not cancel out the other. God is about *balance* in all things. Our job is to try our best to become *like* him so we can return to live *with* him. He gives us the opportunity to change and do better, to *become* better. Paul tells the saints: don't worry about what others are doing, worry about yourself. God will take them who violate his laws into his own hand. [48]

You can't have joy if you are overwhelmed with too much grief, pain, or misery. Likewise, you can't feel peacefully joyful if you are manically excited either. Too much of either is equally harmful. Excess is the enemy just as much as poverty, deficiency, and lack.

There are different triggers that will try to drag us back into our old patterns, those ways we *used* to deal with things. We need to become keenly aware of them so we recognize when we need to ask for support to help get us through that tough time of excess. [49] Extra stress, extra pain, sorrow, insecurities, feeling scared, and maybe a lot of self-doubt. When we are getting lost deep in despair, we are moving further away from being able to feel the very spirit that can nourish us back to health and balance.

This nourishment of spirit is the very thing we need to consume in large quantities to get us back to neutral. When I say "spirit," I'm *not* referring to the false substitute that extreme zealots often resort to. Christ did not approve of those people. I'm saying: consume *the Spirit* frequently and regularly until you get caught up, and then consume at maintenance levels. It's like when you get sick and you eat soup: if you only have one bowl a week until you get better, it's going to take a long time. If you have three bowls of soup a day (and maybe have it for your snacks too), your recovery time will be shortened up quite a lot!

Once we obtain the desired goal of wellness, we cannot stop there. We must *continue* nourishing ourselves and those around us to prevent falling again so deeply. Ignore what those not on the same path say about what you eat—and—when, where, and why. There will be critics, and unfortunately, they will be loud and possibly hateful in their attempts to sway you away from your destination and weaken your determination.

This is why being a part of a like-minded community with which you can regularly spend time is so important— so that you can live and support each other. Watch out for people who say that no one should eat certain foods. Know this: all foods were created to be received with thanksgiving by those who believe and know the truth. [50]

The vineyard of the Lord of Hosts is the house of Israel, God says, and his pleasant plants are the men of Judah. Though he looks here and there for judgment, all he can find is oppression. There's no righteousness, only crying. He warns those plotting evil, even those who plot evil upon themselves. When morning is light, they practice evil because they have power to do so. These people covet lands and houses and take them by violence, oppressing every man, woman, and child; even oppressing their homes and taking away their heritage.

Many houses will be desolate, and many great cities will become uninhabited. There will be famine and starvation. The wine in their feasts, being consumed, without considering the Creator's hand in all things. His people are in captivity simply because they don't have knowledge to free themselves. Their honorable men are famished, and the people are fried up with thirst.

This vineyard represents God's chosen people, who the Bible references as being the nation of Israel. As such, God has cultivated and cared for them very much like a farmer tends to his vineyard and who expects fruitfulness and obedience. The men of Judah, who are the pleasant plants referenced above, are part of the twelve tribes of Israel. Judah was one of the groups who did not fall away after false gods. The northern ten tribes fell away, became scattered, and lost. The little tribe of Benjamin joined and became part of the tribe of Judah. Judah was considered as favored and chosen amongst the Israelites due to their obedience and fruitfulness.

A healthy diet for our body can bring the same kind of results like an obedient and fruitful vineyard. The vineyard is our body and we, the farmer. As we tend, care for, and cultivate our bodies through healthy eating and thinking, it can produce wonderful fruit and become our favored and chosen body, mind, and spirit. Much like the opposite, if we do not tend to it or fill it with garbage and junk, letting it go through drought and improper nourishment, it goes to weed, dries up, and dies. We would find, much like God did when he looked around, only to find bad judgments and only oppression.

When we do not follow the laws of health, we will run into disappointment and frustration. Sometimes we may find rogue plants that are hard to kill growing in our garden. Despite God's best, highest intentions, the vineyard of Israel and Judah did not produce the fruit that he desired from them. Instead of justice and peace, he found violence and bloodshed. Instead of bounty and vigor of strength God's pleasant plants cry out for help in their distress and desperation. We can be like them or we can make a conscious choice every day, to try to become a healthful, fruitful garden.

Taking a look at the lack of justice or judgment we find that there is a lack of fairness and righteousness. This always leads, if not eventually, to suffering, distress, and yes, even crying and oppression. I've definitely had some times in my life that have felt like this and I'm sure that you can think of some examples in your own life as well.

Oppression is quite a heavy word and the feeling associated with the sound of the word is one that weighs you down in mind or body. According to the American Heritage Dictionary oppress means to keep down by severe and unjust use of *force* or authority. To cause to feel worried or depressed. To overwhelm or *crush.* Merriam-Webster's dictionary adds to crush or burden by *abuse of power* or authority. Britannica Dictionary says it's a way of treating a person or group of people in a cruel or unfair way. Strong's Concordance suggests that the word relates to violence, injustice, or cruelty. Do you wield this weapon against others or even yourself in relation to nourishment or health? *Food* for thought.

It may be that many of us have grown up under the hand of oppression of well-meaning parents. We may have learned, incorrectly, that this is how you get things done. Perhaps even, it could be used as a method of self-preservation and protection from those around us. But like using a butter knife to chop down a tree is not the right tool for the job, oppression is not the right way to get to where you need to go. There's a much better tool for any of those jobs and oppression is never one of them for it. Even oppression used with the *intent* to force others to do good, is still used unwisely and is inappropriate. Instead, we need to look within ourselves and find the broken pieces that are wanting us to use this tool, and fix the brokenness within us instead. Surprisingly, if we do this, we suddenly no longer need to oppress others or ourselves. We'll be much happier and healthier in the process. It can be difficult to find or even see that we have these broken places within us ourselves. This is when and why we should seek professional help to find and to heal them. Once we do, what we truly desire, becomes ours or the need no longer exists for why we thought we needed it.

When there is an absence of righteousness in our life, our community, our health, our bodies we will always find that there is a moral and ethical imbalance. There is a lack of respect when it comes to the rights and dignity of an individual. In this case, to ourselves. In what ways are we exacting this type of lawlessness upon our diets, our bodies with the foods we are choosing to put in them? What kinds of thoughts are we feeding our minds, and types of spiritual food are we putting into our souls? When we neglect these things, the overall spirit we will possess will be one of sadness, pain, and despair. The rates of anxiety and depression in these times we live in currently, are shockingly high. We need not look much further than these areas to see why these rates are so incredibly high.

Some people may be guilty of using food as a way of punishing or harming themselves. Whether it is through eating too much of the wrong things or eating too little of the right ones, the intent can be the same. The harm to the body can also result in the same type of despair and destitution. Just as much as someone who intentionally plans and schemes evil against another person we can be just as guilty and accountable for harming ourselves even if it is not something that we are doing consciously. We don't get a free pass for not seeking out solutions or becoming consciously aware. We are held to the same standard either way. We must seek out, learn, and then do the right things and for the right reasons. It won't be overnight or instantaneous results but we *must* try and we must *begin* and then we have to keep trying!

We can spend all night thinking up ways to succeed, to become more healthy, to find new solutions to reach our healthy food goals or we can sleep away slothfully or even go so far as to waste away thinking up new ways to spoil and destroy our own health, our own vineyard. When the morning is light, and we have received our strength from resting all night, this is the precise instant we must stand up and stand for something better for ourselves, our bellies, our bodies and our minds, and for our lives. You have the power to do so, within you. It's in there. You may have to dig deeper to find it or you may have to build up that self-empowerment muscle within you but I promise you, it's there. *Find* it! And then, start using it. *Regularly.*

We may like to believe that we do not covet lands and houses until there is no place left for anyone to live or grow their own food, [51] and yet we need not look farther than to see how we oppress or covet other people's bodies and the appearance of good health in them that we do not see in ourselves. We would take their hard work and accomplishment of good health by violence and we do this in punishing ourselves with bad food choices, bad thoughts, bad behaviors (things that harm us and others) or even against them directly and indirectly. This can appear in the form of shaming others or ourselves. We can

286

oppress others and ourselves in various ways as well. We can expend just as much energy, less even, and wind up with the results we covet in others, for ourselves without stealing from someone else, taking away from them. But we must also do these good health building activities for the right reason, or it will all be wasted.

When we do not eat to nourish our bodies, which are the houses of our spirits, then they become desolate. They can become so sick and depleted that like the many cities that will become uninhabited in our future days, so too have and do many people's bodies become. Empty. Uninhabited.

When we do not eat to nourish, there is famine and starvation within the body. Like attracts like. As an example, a famine is going to attract more famine. How is this? In the literal sense, in a famine, there is no water and plants die. Plants help to hold water and moisture in the soil which helps keep more plants alive and trapping a larger area of water in the soil.

Have you ever noticed an empty field that has nothing but a small seed starting to grow in it? Eventually over time, it reproduces, sends out suckers which help to shade the ground around the original plant and attract more moisture. It also helps to cool the air temperature right in that area. As more of that one plant grows, more things will also start to thrive there until suddenly it seems that the whole field is covered in growing things. This also begins to attract insects and animals who depend on these things to stay alive. They in turn leave fertilizer for the plants through their waste which strengthens the soil and soon you have an entire ecosystem in place. It all started with one little seed and the tiniest little bit of water and natural sunlight.

Starvation attracts more starvation. By natural laws, we become absolutely and literally consumed through a lack of consumption. This is highly ironic. As we suffer from a lack of food, and are hungry to the point that there is suffering from deprivation, the body becomes less and less able to absorb other nutrients even if they are readily available in the body. As we do not provide the things needed to create more energy, it is forced to consume itself, a sort of cannibalism or catabolysis, if you will. The muscles begin to atrophy in order to stay alive. The process is the breaking down of the body's own muscle tissue to obtain energy and nutrients during times of severe malnutrition, starvation, or chronic illness. Signs you may recognize in this are things like low energy levels, exercise intolerance, reduced ability to handle stress, and wasting away. None of these are healthy for the body, mind, or spirit and are very dangerous when maintained over an extended period of time.

We must remember and consider that the Creator made all these things like plants, and animals for us, even our bodies, and we should show our thankfulness by remembering to be grateful for them. How and why these things were created are miraculous and truly marvelous! If it were easy, everyone would be doing it, of course. All of creation was made for us to use them in wisdom and order. When we do so they bring us life and fullness and we absolutely thrive. And, when we don't, we get the opposite: death, depression, and frailty. Gratitude is key to all things that nourish and fill us up.

The reference to the wine being consumed at the feasts without acknowledging the Creator's role in their lives refers us to a gaping black hole within us seeking to be filled with something. It will remain insatiable until it is filled, however, with the thing that it needs and desires most. It is our job to fill it with the right things and avoiding the wrong things. Whether we realize this or not, this lack of awareness and appreciation affects us in more ways than we may have first imagined. When this lack exists it leads to a kind of captivity with us. This comes from our own lack of knowledge. Lack of knowledge is ignorance and ignorance of this type is gross and inexcusable. Let me explain.

Ignorance is bliss! Who knew such a little thing as ignorance could be so entailed *and* so deceptive? It sounds so cheerful, happy even when you say it, or when you hear it repeated in jest. You can't say it without smiling! And just like the lie that it is, it has a false face to go with it. What do I mean? I think many people get the sense of false security when they hear this phrase and relax into a state of feeling this excuses them from even trying. All is well. And so, they skip along their merry way down the path of life, blissful and ignorant.

However, what ignorance keeps distracting people from, like a child with an all-day-sucker, is the growing debt of responsibilities and harm to themselves and others that is mounting along behind and beside them. They ignore the rising tide of grief and pain around them as the thunder clouds rumble louder and lower overhead. Yet as long as they stay focused on their ignorance-sucker, they like to believe the world is sunny and filled with rainbows and daisies.

The word ignorance in the GNU version of the Collaborative International Dictionary of English has basically three definitions. There's the general sense of ignorance. This means that you basically lack knowledge in general in relation to a given subject or are basically uneducated or uninformed. I think *most* of us like to stop there in relation to understanding the term. But we must delve deeper into the *meaning* of this word, because it's important to understand it fully and be able to move on.

Ignorance also means to have a *willful* neglect or *refusal* to acquire knowledge which one *may* acquire and it is his *duty* to have. [*italics added for emphasis*] Now, this is an entirely different animal in my perspective and I think many of us fall under this category and definition of the word ignorant, whether we'd like to admit it to ourselves or not. Especially living in a full-access through technology world, there is no limit to the information that we can dig up, research, and find. Really, there is no reason not to do it so that definitely makes it willful and a refusal to seek out greater knowledge, light, and understanding on a topic.

The third definition of ignorance is the type that is *beyond* a person's individual *control* and that which we are *not* responsible to God for. I think a lot of us like to confuse the second definition for this one. We like to think and tell ourselves it's out of our control and allow ourselves permission to give up and just not go looking believing our definition of justice will be fine. However, God has said *that* is not the standard he is using for us. We *will* be held responsible for the knowledge we seek to obtain *and* what we *do not* seek for in this life. Only he can know which is which and we are far better off working off the second definition than hoping we can skate by with this last one. We cannot say, we'll only be judged for what we know so I won't go looking. We are and will be accountable whether we even know we'll be or not. In other words, we will be accountable for the *not* looking as much as for what we *did* look for and maybe even more so. What we did with our knowledge also matters.

Some may make the mistake of thinking there's no harm in remaining ignorant and that it won't hurt anyone but themselves. Perhaps they haven't seemed to notice the repercussions at all or yet. However, it is important to understand the gravity that the lack of knowledge leads a person into captivity.

When you do not know or understand things you are easily fooled and beguiled even to the point that truth could be placed before you and you not even recognize it. You may even ridicule and mock those who have knowledge, making yourself look the fool instead whether you realize it or not. Then your ignorance becomes very transparent to those with knowledge and they see your "knowledge nakedness" so to speak. Having others join you in ignorantly ridiculing those with knowledge does not make you any less "knowledge naked" to those who know. It only allows you to cling desperately to that ignorance-sucker a little bit longer. The darkness inches closer and closer and your fake daisy world of sunshine and rainbows dissolves away. If instead, you embraced knowledge, you would keep all the darkness and gloom at bay and be able to live in a real world where you could create lasting sunshine and rainbows. False worlds and lives are like living in starvation. It truly doesn't feel good. This is why normally honorable men are famished and the people experiencing extreme thirst. There is a massive level of suffering and desperation. People are seeking the answers yet not knowing where to turn. But we *must* turn. We must *look*. And, we *must* see and then *do*. Having truth and full nourishment are the way to go, to thrive, to be zestfully alive!

All things are restored through Christ. He did away with the old laws because they were fulfilled in him on the cross. Those laws were needed to teach Israel to fulfill all righteousness, to live holy and clean lives. He came to begin the *restoration* of the *fulness* of the law that had been lost. God teaches us line upon line. A little instruction here, and little knowledge and experience there. It's not a destination. It's a *journey*. Much like a ladder to completeness, it must be climbed one foot, a hand, and then one step at a time. You can't skip to the end or jump ahead. You must master and become an expert at each rung of the ladder. For most of us, we'll have to climb that ladder multiple times. *Ugh...*I don't even want to *think* about how many times *I* will have to climb it over again with my many imperfections. Thank goodness for do-overs and U-turns!

I need help sometimes. Realistically, I should say I need help all the time! Everyone does, and there's no shame in saying it. There are times I just don't know what to do, and sometimes I'm so overwhelmed I can't find my way through the chaos and noise that's clamoring to be heard. Food has been my comfort; it has been my solace, my protection at times, and my friend when I felt so alone. Food has *also* been my great enemy and prison guard.

How can food be my friend and can it be a good one? To choose our friends wisely, we must first know ourselves.

Our strengths and weaknesses are essential knowledge to have about ourselves when we begin any journey. We must have our pillar of priorities in place. A pillar in the wrong place can block your path at best and make your structure unstable or collapse at worst. Also having pillars made out of strong stable and reliable principles or nutrients is a must! We must know the difference between right and wrong, deception and clarity, might and will. *And,* we must understand how they all relate to food.

Things that are right about nutrition include growing and eating foods that are local, 100% organic, clean, and healthy. It's right to want—even demand!—these things. We must realize that not everyone on this planet is our friend. Not everyone is looking out for our best interests.

Therefore, we must look for and find those who think, feel, and believe similarly (in respect to foods) and work together with those people to create a better living environment. That does *not* mean everyone has to think exactly the same, just similarly as to mutual respect. And these people who we work with must respect and be willing to listen to differences and take the time to listen and understand. Not to hear only, but to *listen* and *understand.*

Food gives us strength. When used properly, it gives us hope, passion, and a zeal for life. When *not* used properly, it has the opposite effect. It can deaden our emotions, burden our internal systems unnecessarily, and lead to overload and overwhelm. If you let it, the world will lead you to believe your body can handle a lot more on a daily basis than it was meant to handle.

We need to learn to treat our bodies more gently and be a lot easier on them. We must be mindful of the things we are taking into our bodies, whether it's the shows that we watch, the music to which we listen, the language we choose to use when we communicate, and the conversations that we have with other people. We need to be much more respectful and kinder to ourselves regarding the things entering and leaving our bodies and minds.

What we feed our mind and our senses can have a detrimental effect if we are not watchful and careful about what input we receive. We will struggle to make up our minds, figure out how we feel about things, and end up not having the coping skills we need to thrive naturally. Instead, it will all end up in the garbage dump: jumbled, complex, and a hot mess. We need to know ourselves from the inside out, all the parts. If we can do that, we will be well on our way to finding the balance in our lives that we've been looking for, hoping for, and dreaming of.

Foods Tree of Paradise


~~~
~~~

References

(King James Version of the Bible unless otherwise noted.)

CHAPTER 1
* Telomere – repetitive DNA sequences at the ends of chromosomes that protect them from becoming frayed or tangled (like the plastic tips at the end of shoelaces, but for DNA)
1. 1 Corinthians 8:3
** psychologytoday.com/us/basics/cognitive-dissonance
2. 1 Thessalonians 5:6
3. 2 Kings 20:1
4. Matthew 4:23
Figure 1. The Wellness Triangle

CHAPTER 2
5. Psalms 103:3
6. Genesis 8:20
*** departments.washington.edu
**** firesafetysupport.com
7. Galatians 5:21
+ National Institute on Alcohol Abuse and Alcoholism: niaaa.nih.gov/alcohols-effects-health/alcohols-effects-body
8. Titus 1:7
++ *Prevention Magazine*
9. Matthew 8:14
10. John 4:53
11. Acts 28:8

CHAPTER 3

12. Genesis 1:29
13. 1 Samuel 14:24
14. Psalms 78:25
15. James 2:15
16. Luke 13:11
17. Exodus 4:6
18. 2 Kings 5:1
Strong's Concordance: biblestudytools.com/concordances/strongs-exhaustive-concordance/
19. Colossians 2:16
20. Isaiah 25:4
21. Exodus 23:25
22. Acts 24:25
23. Galatians 5:23
24. 1 Peter 4:3
25. Daniel 1:8
26. Matthew 9:17
27. 1 Timothy 3:3
28. 1 Kings 3:28

CHAPTER 4

29. Acts 6:10
30. Proverbs 3:8

CHAPTER 5

31. Isaiah 6:10, Acts 28:27
32. Genesis 1:29
33. Genesis 9:3,10-14
34. Leviticus 10:9
35. Numbers 6:3
36. Deuteronomy 14:3

37. Proverbs 3:8
38. Proverbs 20:1
39. Proverbs 23:2
40. Proverbs 23:21
41. Ecclesiastes 10:17
42. Isaiah 5:22
43. Isaiah 24:9
44. Isaiah 28:7
45. Daniel 1:8
46. Habakkuk 2:15
47. 1 Corinthians 3:17
48. 1 Corinthians 6:10
49. Ephesians 5:18
50. 1 Timothy 4:3
51. Isaiah 5:8, Micah 2:2

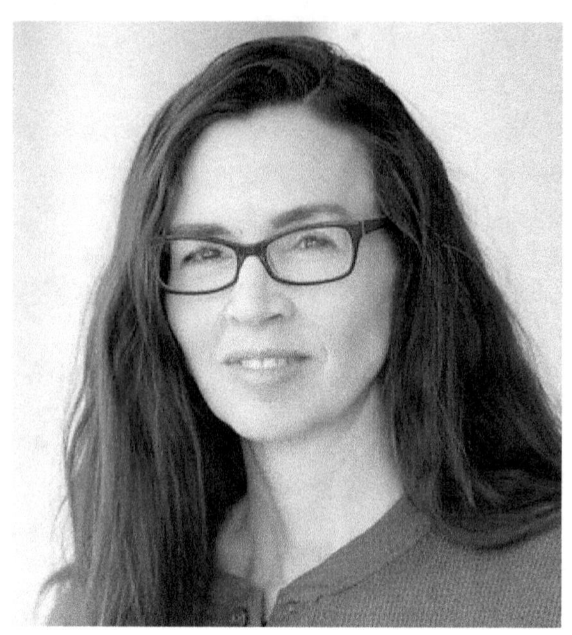

R. Shelton, CLMT, BCTMB

R. Shelton is a licensed and board-certified bodyworker, wellness provider, and award-winning nonfiction author. She specializes in clinically styled bodywork of many varieties. Shelton is dedicated to results and being an example of wellness for her clients. She loves learning new things, cooking tasty recipes and eating them, dance, music, time with loved ones, and serving in her community.

Post Your Book Review

Did you enjoy the material or learn something new? How did reading *Food's Tree of Paradise* impact you? Share your thoughts by leaving a heartfelt review where you bought the book.

Post stars. It's a quick and easy way to thank an author for their hard work so they write more.

Want to write a review people will find helpful and love to read? The best ones are detailed and specific. Think: How did it make you feel? What do you want to change in your life now? Get a little personal and touch on points that other readers will find helpful too. What did you relate to? Aim for 100-150 words and break up paragraphs into 2-3 sentences for easier reading.

(If you find any typos or mistakes, don't put those in your review! Instead, feel free to contact me or the publisher directly about those so we can correct them. It's impossible to catch everything, even with a team of professionals looking at it, but with your help we can find them all!)

I look forward to reading *your* review! – R. Shelton

Book Recommended For:

Corporate Wellness Plans

School or University Use for Departments Of:

- Behavioral Science and Human Services

- Exercise Science

- Fitness

- Health Science

- Psychology

- Wellness Education

Class Resource Acquisitions

Book Clubs

Church Groups

Retail Stores

Health and Wellness Centers

And More

NOTE: If interested in using the book for a specific class or program, ask about the <u>How to Teach using Member Heal Thyself</u> manuals created for educators and provider specific user manuals for licensed and certified use. They are available online or you may order physical copies if approved.

Also by R. Shelton:

1. Member Heal Thyself
2. Fountain of Living Water
3. Food's Tree of Paradise
4. coming soon...

Member Heal Thyself

A much-needed book of life instructions for healing ourselves naturally. A resource that guides us to use the full potential of our physical bodies.

Fountain of Living Water

Supplemental to the book, *Member Heal Thyself,* that reviewers showered with praises. Readers requested that the author create more thirst-quenching information on the topic of hydration.

This book covers the first of "*Member Heal Thyself's*" twelve resources; "Hydration" much more in depth and in all its various aspects including many surprising details not covered in the first book.

- Discover mysteries: missing healing properties of water and the impacts on every drop of life.

- Be inspired: historical analogies narratively sprinkled through touching vulnerability, explore new ways to use water never before dreamed of

- Be changed: tailor steps to preferred personal needs with nature's natural resource.

Drink your fill to overflowing!

Upcoming book: title TBA...

Supplemental to the book that reviewers showered with praises, *Member Heal Thyself*. Readers requested that we create more heart-pumping information on the topic of exercise.

This book covers the third of "*Member Heal Thyself's*" twelve resources; "Exercise" much more in depth and in all its various aspects including many surprising details not covered in the first book.

- Discover mysteries: missing healing properties of exercise and the impacts on every muscle, gland, and cell in the body.

- Be inspired: historical analogies narratively sprinkled through touching vulnerability, explore new ways to use exercise never before dreamed of

- Be changed: tailor steps to preferred personal needs in harmony with the body's natural movements.

Get pumped!

Contact Us at:

info@memberhealthyself.com

for information regarding large purchase orders.